Nursing as Caring
A Model for Transforming Practice

Nursing as Caring
A Model for Transforming Practice

Anne Boykin
Savina Schoenhofer

National League for Nursing Press • New York
Pub. No. 15-2549

ISBN 0-88737-601-0

Library of Congress Cataloging-in-Publication Data

Boykin, Anne
   Nursing as caring : a model for transforming practice / Anne Boykin, Savina Schoenhofer.
     p.   cm.
   "Pub. no. 15-2549."
   Includes bibliographical references and index.
   ISBN 0-88737-601-0 : $35.00
   1. Nursing—Philosophy. 2. Caring. I. Schoenhofer, Savina O'Bryan. II. Title.
   [DNLM: 1. Empathy. 2. Nursing Theory. 3. Models, Nursing. WY 86 B791n 1993]
RT84.5.B69   1993
610.73'01—dc20
DNLM/DLC
for Library of Congress   93-23021
                                          CIP

CONTENTS

ABOUT THE AUTHORS

Anne Boykin, PhD, is Dean, College of Nursing, Florida Atlantic University, Boca Raton, Florida. She is President of the International Association for Human Caring, a former member of the NLN Board of Review, is active in the American Association of Colleges of Nursing, a member of the Board of Directors of Southern Council on Collegiate Education in Nursing, and numerous regional and state organizations. Dr. Boykin is an internationally known consultant for nursing education. She has published widely on caring in nursing.

Savina Schoenhofer, PhD, is Graduate Program Director, College of Nursing, Florida Atlantic University, Boca Raton, Florida. She is co-founder of *Nightingale Songs*, a publication of nurses' stories. Dr. Schoenhofer established the Nursing Research Development Network, a collaboration of nurses in practice and education settings which has created an agenda for regional nursing research. Her publications have been in the areas of nursing home management, nursing values, caring, and touch as a medium for nursing in critical care settings.

These authors are currently involved in designing an innovative health care delivery model for a comprehensive center for older adults. This effort represents the first opportunity for creating a health care facility grounded in Nursing as Caring.

FOREWORD

*C*aring may be one of the most often used words in the English language. Indeed, the word is commonly used as much in talking about our everyday lives and relationships as it is in the marketplace. At the same time, nurses thinking about, doing, and describing nursing know that caring has unique and particular meaning to them. Caring is one of the first synonyms for nursing offered by nursing students and is surely the most frequent word used by the public in talking about nursing. Caring is an essential value in the personal and professional lives of nurses. The formal recognition of caring in nursing as an area of study and as a necessary guide for the various avenues of nursing practice, however, is relatively new. Anne Boykin and Savina Schoenhofer have received many requests from academic peers and students to articulate the nursing theory they have been working to develop. This book is a response to the call for a theory of nursing as caring.

The progression of nursing theory development often has been led by nurse theorists who stepped into other disciplines for ways to think about and study nursing and for structures and concepts to describe nursing practice. The opportunity to use language and methods of familiar, relatively established bodies of knowledge that could be communicated and widely understood took shape as many nursing scholars received graduate education in disciplines outside of nursing. Conceptions and methods of knowledge development often came then from disciplines in the biological and social sciences and were brought into ways of thinking about and doing nursing scholarship. Evolution of new worldviews opened the way for nurses to develop theories reflecting ideas of energy fields, wholeness, processes, and patterns. Working from outside the discipline of nursing, along with shifts in worldviews, has been essential to opening the way for nurses to explore nursing as a unique practice and body of knowledge from inside the discipline, and to know nursing in unprecedented ways.

Nursing as Caring: A Model for Transforming Practice sets forth a different order of nursing theory. This nursing theory is personal, not abstract. In order to express nursing as caring there is a clear need to know self as caring person. The focus of the Nursing as Caring theory, then, is not toward an end product such as health or wellness. It is about a unique way of living caring in the world. It is about nurses and nursed living life and nurturing growing humanly through participation in life together.

Nursing as caring sets forth nursing as a unique way of living caring in the world. This theory provides a view that can be lived in all nursing situations and can be practiced alone or in combination with other theories. The domain of nursing is nurturing caring. The integrity, the wholeness, and the connectedness of the person simply and assuredly is central. As such, this is perhaps the most basic, bedrock, and therefore radical, of nursing theories and is essential to all that is truly nursing.

The dynamic, living idea of nursing as caring must be expressed knowledgeably. Perhaps for this reason, the book presents the essence of the idea and encourages its careful study and understanding in full hope for further development. In this regard, many questions come to mind in thinking about this work and its importance for the discipline and practice of nursing.

- What distinguishes this nursing theory from others?
- In what ways does this work add to the body of nursing knowledge?
- In what new and distinct ways are we to view theories of our discipline and practice?
- What are new descriptions of processes for development, study, and appraisal of nursing theories?
- How will new relationships among nursing theories be discovered and described?

As earlier theorists brought words and ways of other bodies of knowledge to help nurses know and articulate nursing, so some of the language of this new theory has been drawn from philosophy. Generally, the language used to express the theory of nursing as caring is everyday language. This model is a clear assertion of and for nursing—it distinguishes nursing knowledge, questions, and methods from those of other disciplines. It helps us explore ways to use nursing knowledge and knowledge of other disciplines in ways appropriate to nursing. This volume offers rich illustrations of nursing that will immediately seem familiar to most nurses. Many nurses will come to know new possibilities for nursing practice, teaching, administration, and inquiry more fully.

In trying to open the door of this book and invite the reader to explore the Nursing as Caring model, I am personally aware that the living of nursing and the commitment nursing calls forth cannot be fully measured. Each of us is part of the ongoing creation of nursing as we share our experience of nursing. These attempts to share our nursing are a major part of the development of nursing as a discipline and professional practice. Our expressions about nursing are continually challenged as part of the creating process.

The processes of theory development have been the ongoing gift of many nursing scholars, theorists, and researchers. In expressing this new theory of Nursing as Caring, nurses have again courageously stepped forward to develop, articulate, and publish ideas that seem very new to many, and in doing so have risked to offer opportunity for a full range of responses to this work. I know Anne Boykin and Savina Schoenhofer invite with great anticipation responses from nurses and will appreciate opportunity for dialogue.

Marilyn E. Parker, PhD, RN
Associate Professor of Nursing
Florida Atlantic University
Boca Raton, FL

PREFACE

*T*he ideas which led to the development of the theory of Nursing as Caring have their beginnings in our personal histories and came together when we met in 1983. As we participated in the work of establishing nursing as an academic discipline and creating a nursing curriculum grounded in caring at Florida Atlantic University, each of us learned to value the special insights brought by the other. We also discovered early on that we shared a deep devotion to nursing—to the idea of nursing, to the practice of nursing, to the development of nursing.

Several years ago, we realized that our thinking had developed to the extent that we were working with more than a concept. Although we are well aware of an ongoing debate in nursing over technical versus philosophical connotations of theory, we characterize our work as a general theory of nursing developed in the context of our understanding of human science. While we are familiar with the formal concept of theory used in disciplines grouped in the physical and natural sciences, we believe that mathematical form is not an appropriate model for theory work in the discipline of nursing. Therefore, we do not present our work in the traditional form of concepts, definitions, statements, and propositions, but have struggled to find ways to preserve the integrity of nursing as caring through our expressions.

Our thinking has been particularly influenced by the work of two scholars, Mayeroff and Roach. Both of these authors have given voice to caring in important ways—Mayeroff in terms of generic caring, and Roach in terms of caring person as well as caring in nursing. We are aware of other influences on our understanding of caring and caring in nursing, including Paterson and Zderad, Watson, Ray, Leininger, and Gaut. Our conception of nursing as a discipline has been directly influenced by Phenix, King and Brownell, and the Nursing Development Conference Group. While this is not an exhaustive listing of the scholars who have contributed to the development of our ideas, we have made a deliberate effort to review the evolution of our thinking and to recognize significant specific contributions.

Chapter 1 presents a discussion of key ideas that ground and contextualize nursing as caring. The most fundamental idea is that of person as caring with nursing conceptualized as a discipline. Our understanding of this foundation has been seasoned both from within nursing and from outside the discipline, but always with the purpose of deepening our understanding of nursing. When we have gone outside the discipline to extend possibilities for understanding, we have made an effort to go beyond application, to think through the nursing relevance of ideas that seemed, on the surface, to be useful. Chapter 1 and subsequent chapters draw on Mayeroff's (1971) caring ingredients, including:

- Knowing—Explicitly and implicitly, knowing that and knowing how, knowing directly and knowing indirectly (p. 14).

- Alternating rhythm—Moving back and forth between a narrower and a wider framework, between action and reflection (p. 15).

- Patience—Not a passive waiting but participating with the other, giving fully of ourselves (p. 17).

- Honesty—Positive concept that implies openness, genuineness, and seeing truly (p. 18).

- Trust—Trusting the other to grow in his or her own time and own way (p. 20).

- Humility—Ready and willing to learn more about other and self and what caring involves (p. 23).

- Hope—"An expression of the plenitude of the present, alive with a sense of a possible" (p. 26).

- Courage—Taking risks, going into the unknown, trusting (p. 27).

In Chapter 2, we present the theory in its most general form. We have resisted the temptation to include examples in this chapter for two reasons: first, because an example always seemed to lead to the need to further explain and illustrate; and second, because we wished to have a general expression of the theory, undelimited by particulars, and available to facilitate further theory development.

Chapter 3 elaborates on the idea of the nursing situation, and illustrates the practical meaning of the theory in a range of particular nursing situations. This chapter will probably be most satisfying to the reader whose everyday nursing discourse is that of nursing practice. Some might find it useful to read this chapter first, before reading Chapters 1 and 2.

In Chapter 4, we explore the practice of nursing as caring and discuss nursing service administration from the perspective of the theory. Chapter 5 addresses issues and strategies for transforming nursing education and nursing education administration based on nursing as caring.

Our understanding of nursing as a human science discipline is the central focus of Chapter 6. In this chapter, we discuss the necessity of transforming modes of nursing inquiry to facilitate the further development of nursing knowledge in the context of the theory of Nursing as Caring. We also share our commitment to the ongoing development of nursing as caring and directions we wish to take in living that commitment.

It has been our intention to organize and communicate the initial, comprehensive presentation of Nursing as Caring usefully for nurses in practice, as well as those in administrative and academic roles. We have benefited wonderfully from the dialogue resulting from formal and informal opportunities to share this work as it evolved. We look forward to continuing the dialogue.

Anne Boykin, PhD
Dean
College of Nursing
Florida Atlantic University
Boca Raton, FL

Savina Schoenhofer, PhD
Graduate Program Director
College of Nursing
Florida Atlantic University
Boca Raton, FL

REFERENCES

Mayeroff, M. (1971). *On Caring*. New York: Harper & Row.

INTRODUCTION

*T*he study of human caring as a unique and essential characteristic of nursing practice has gradually expanded from early definitional, philosophical, and cultural research on the meanings of caring, to the explication of theoretical definitions of caring, conceptual models, proposed taxonomy of caring concepts, a great deal of creative experimentation with research methodologies, and the development of several theories of caring.

In general, one may say that knowledge of caring has grown in two ways, first by extension and, more recently, by intension. Growth by extension consists in a relatively full explanation of a small region which is then carried over into an explanation of adjoining regions. Growth by extension can be associated with the metaphors of building a model or putting together a jigsaw puzzle (Kaplan, 1964, p. 305).

In growth by intension, a partial explanation of a whole region is made more and more adequate and outlines for subsequent theory and observation are clarified. Growth by intension is associated with the metaphor of gradually illuminating a darkened room. A few persons enter the room with their individual lights and are able to slowly perceive what is in that room. As more persons enter the room, it becomes more fully illuminated, and the observed reality is clarified (Kaplan, 1964, p. 305).

Growth by extension is implicit in the early caring definitions, explications, and models. The knowledge about caring was built up piece-by-piece, in the first ten years of study, by a few nurse scholars committed to the study of human care and caring.

Today, some fifteen years later, progress in the study of the caring phenomenon is no longer piecemeal but gradual and on a larger scale, with illumination from the works that have preceded. Growth by intension is evidenced by the development of an extant bibliography, categorization of caring conceptualizations, and the further development of human care/caring theories. Although the concept of caring has not been definitively and exhaustively explored, the understanding of the broad-scale phenomena of human care and caring has become enlarged. A review of the caring literature by Smerke (1989) and an analysis of the nursing research on care and caring by Morse, Bottoroff, Neander, and Solberg (1990) now provides researchers with an interdisciplinary guide to human caring literature and a categorization of five major conceptualizations of caring: (1) a human trait, (2) a moral imperative, (3) an affect, (4) an interpersonal interaction, and (5) an intervention. There is now a body of knowledge about care and caring that can be used to further develop new knowledge through subsequent theory and research.

The Boykin and Schoenhofer work, *Nursing as Caring: A Model for Transforming Practice,* is an excellent example of growth by intension. Utilizing previous caring research, caring theory, and personal knowledge, the authors have put forth a theory that will not only increase the content of caring knowledge but will also change its form. A new theory adds some knowledge and it transforms what was previously known, clarifying it and giving it new meaning as well as more confirmation. The whole structure of caring knowledge changes with growth, even though it is recognizably similar to what it has been. As one reads this theory, many of the assumptions presented seem familiar, perhaps because the authors realized that caring theory could best be understood in both its historical and immediate context.

The historical context of the systematic study, explication, and theorizing about human care and caring phenomena in nursing began some twenty years ago with the early work of Madeleine Leininger. The first structural stones were laid by a group of nurse researchers who met for the first time in 1978 at a conference convened by Dr. Leininger at the University of Utah in Salt Lake City. Some sixteen enthusiastic participants underscored the need for continued in-depth thinking and for sharing scholarly ideas about the phenomena and nature of caring.

Plans were made to continue with yearly research conferences focused on four major goals:

1. The identification of major philosophical, epistemological, and professional dimensions of caring to advance the body of knowledge that constitutes nursing.

2. Explication of the nature, scope, and functions of caring and its relationship to nursing care.

3. Explication of the major components, processes, and patterns of care or caring in relationship to nursing care from a transcultural perspective.

4. Stimulation of nurse scholars to systematically investigate care and caring and to share their findings with others.

These four goals, developed by the members of the Caring Research Conference Group, provided nurse scholars with a direction for caring research that yielded a substantial piece of research-based literature.

The first ten years of the Conference group (1978–1988) witnessed a great deal of diverse and stimulating research. Major philosophical dimensions of caring were explicated in the works of Bevis (1981), Gaut (1984), Gustafson (1984), Ray (1981), Roach (1984), and Watson (1979).

Explication of major components, processes, and patterns of care or caring from a transcultural perspective was first developed in the early work of Aamodt (1978) and Leininger (1978, 1981), to be followed by the works of Baziak-Dugan (1984), Boyle (1984), Guthrie (1981), Wang (1984), and Wenger and Wenger (1988).

Another group of nurse researchers chose to study the concept of care and caring concomitantly with nursing care practices. Brown (1982), Gardner and Wheeler (1981), Knowlden (1985), Larson (1981, 1984), Riemen (1984, 1986), Sherwood (1991), and Wolf (1986) investigated nurse behaviors perceived by patients and nurses as indicators of caring and noncaring in an attempt to further develop the essential structure of a caring interaction.

Watson, Burckhardt, Brown, Block, and Hester (1979) proposed an alternative health care model for nursing practice and research. After seven years of implementation experience using a clinical practice model with various hospitals, Wesorick (1990) presented a model that supported caring as a practice norm in hospital settings.

Administrative caring within an institutional or organizational culture was the research focus for Nyberg (1989), Ray (1984, 1989), Valentine (1989, 1991), and Wesorick (1990, 1991). Caring within educational settings and in the teacher–learner relationship also received attention by Bevis (1978), Bush (1988), Condon (1986), and MacDonald (1984).

Introduction

Research methodologies became a focus of study as investigators struggled with how best to study nurse caring phenomena: Boyle (1981), Gaut (1981, 1985), Larson (1981), Leininger (1976), Ray (1985), Riemen (1986), Swanson-Kauffman (1986), Valentine (1988), Watson (1985), and Wenger (1985).

By the 1980s, it became clear that the systematic study of human care and caring as a distinct feature of the profession of nursing had evolved globally. Dunlop (1986), from Australia, asked: "Is a science of caring possible?" Bjrn (1987) described the caring sciences in Denmark, and Eriksson (1987, 1992) began to develop her theories of caring as communion, and caring as health. Kleppe (1987) discussed the background and development of caring research in Norway. Flynn (1988) compared the caring communities of nursing in England and the United States. Halldorsdottir (1989, 1991), from Iceland, developed research on caring and uncaring encounters in nursing practice and in nursing education.

The early endeavors of the first nurse researchers who focused on caring laid out the lines and clarified the observable realities for subsequent research and theorizing. The production of nursing theory is dependent on an intellectual apprehension of the movement between the concrete realities of nursing practice and the abstract world of those assumptions and propositions known as theories (Benoliel, 1977, p. 110). The creation of new knowledge rests on some known assumptions, and Boykin and Schoenhofer's theory builds on the work of three other nurse scholars who have developed theories of caring in nursing, each with a differing apprehension of the realities of human care and caring: Madeleine Leininger from an anthropological perspective—one of the first nurse theorists to focus on caring as the essence of nursing practice; Sister M. Simone Roach, who provides a philosophical and theological perspective; and Jean Watson from an existential, philosophical perspective.

The significance of Leininger's Culture-Care Theory (1993) is in the study of human care from a transcultural nursing perspective. This focus has led to new and unique insights about care and the nature of caring and nursing in different cultures, and has developed the knowledge so essential to providing culturally sensitive nursing care throughout the world.

Roach's work, *The Human Act of Caring* (1984, 1992) is recognized as one of the most substantive, insightful, and sensitive publications on human caring. Her ultimate conclusion after years of study and reflection is: "Caring is the human mode of being."

Watson, in her theory of human care (1985, 1989), addressed the issue of nursing as a humanistic science rather than a formal or biological science. This perspective was an essential paradigm shift for nursing knowledge, but essential for study of the caring phenomena. Within this context, Watson developed a theory of caring in nursing that involves values, a will and commitment to care, knowledge, caring actions and consequences. Caring then becomes a moral imperative for practitioners of the profession of nursing.

Boykin and Schoenhofer's theory comes not only from "what is known about caring" but also from their imagination and creative sense of "what could be known." They suggest a context for personal theorizing about caring experiences, trusting that each person will examine the content of those experiences as a sequence of more or less meaningful events— meaningful both in themselves and in the patterns of their occurrence. The authors put forth a framework for just such reflection, and they challenge practicing nurses to "come to know self as caring person in ever deepening and broadening dimensions."

If science has to do with knowing and that which is known, then theory is about knowledge production. In one sense of the term, theory activity might well be regarded as the most important and distinctive for human beings because it stands for the symbolic dimension of experience (Kaplan, 1964, p. 294).

Boykin and Schoenhofer's work invites all nurses to develop nursing knowledge and to theorize from within the nursing situation. The invitation requests a sharing of both content and context of nursing experiences as they are lived in meaningful patterns that have significant bearings on all other patterns. To engage in theorizing means not only to learn *by* experience, but to learn *from* experience—that is, to take thought about what is there to be learned (Kaplan, 1964, p. 295).

In the thinking of Alfred North Whitehead (1967), theory functions not to allow prediction but to provide a frame of reference, a pattern through which one can discern particulars of any given situation. Theory in this sense permits attendance or focus by giving form to otherwise unstructured content. The proposed theory, *Nursing as Caring: A Model for Transforming Practice,* provides the context. The frame of reference through which any nurse engaged in a shared lived experience of caring can not only interpret the experience but also can perceive and symbolically express the patterns of nurse caring. The perception of patterns will give the readers and listeners a "click of meaningfulness," and the explanation will be the discovery of interconnections among patterns. The perception that everything is just where it should be to complete the pattern is what gives us intellectual satisfaction and provides the context or focus for the one aspect of reality that is the essence of nursing-caring.

Delores A. Gaut PhD, RN
Immediate Past President
International Association of Human Caring, Inc.
Visiting Professor
University of Portland School of Nursing
Portland, Oregon

REFERENCES

Aamodt, A. (1978). The care component in a health and healing system (pp. 37–45). In Bauwens (Ed.), *Anthropology and health.* St. Louis: Mosby.

Baziak-Dugan, A. (1984). Compadrazgo: A caring phenomenon among urban Latinos and its relationship to health. In M. Leininger (Ed.), *Care: The essence of nursing and health* (pp. 183–194). Detroit, MI: Wayne State University Press.

Benoliel, J. (1977). The interaction between theory and research. *Nursing Outlook, 25*(2), 108–113.

Bevis, E. (1978). Curriculum building in nursing (2nd ed.). St. Louis: Mosby.

Bevis, E. (1981). Caring: A life force. In M. Leininger, *Caring: An essential human need* (pp. 49–59). Detroit, MI: Wayne State University Press.

Bjrn, A. (1987). Caring sciences in Denmark *Scandinavian Journal of Caring Sciences, 1*(1), 3–6.

Boyle, J. (1981). An application of the structural–functional method to the phenomenon of caring. In M. Leininger (Ed.), *Caring: An essential human need* (pp. 37–47). Detroit, MI: Wayne State University Press.

Introduction

Boyle, J. (1984). Indigenous caring practices in a Guatemalan Colonia. In M. Leininger (Ed.), *Care: The essence of nursing and health* (pp. 123–132). Detroit, MI: Wayne State University Press.

Brown, C. (1991). Caring in nursing administration: Healing through empowering. In D. Gaut & M. Leininger (Eds.), *Caring: The compassionate healer* (pp. 123–134). New York: National League for Nursing.

Brown, L. (1986). The experiences of care: Patient perspectives: *Topics in Clinical Nursing, 8*(2), 56–62.

Bush, H. (1988). The caring teacher of nursing. In M. Leininger (Ed.), *Care: Discovery and uses in clinical and community nursing* (pp. 169–187). Detroit, MI: Wayne State University Press.

Condon, E. (1986). Theory derivation: Application to nursing, the caring perspective within professional role development. *Journal of Nursing Education, 25*(4), 156–159.

Dunlop, M. J. (1986). Is a science of caring possible? *Journal of Advanced Nursing, 11*(6), 661–670.

Eriksson, K. (1987). Pausen. Stockholm: Almqvist & Wiksell.

Eriksson, K. (1992). The alleviation of suffering—the idea of caring. *Scandinavian Journal of Caring Sciences, 6*(2), 119–123.

Flynn, B. C. (1988). The caring community: Primary health care and nursing in England and the United States. In M. Leininger (Ed.), *Care: Discovery and uses in clinical and community nursing* (pp. 29–38). Detroit, MI: Wayne State University Press.

Gardner, K., & Wheeler, E. (1981). The meaning of caring in the context of nursing. In M. Leininger (Ed.), *Caring: An essential human need* (pp. 69–79). Detroit, MI: Wayne State University Press.

Gaut, D. A. (1983). Development of a theoretically adequate description of caring. *Western Journal of Nursing Research, 5*(4), 312–324.

Gaut, D. A. (1984). A theoretic description of caring as action. In M. Leininger (Ed.), *Care: The essence of nursing and health* (pp. 27–44). Detroit, MI: Wayne State University Press.

Gaut, D. A. (1985). Philosophical analysis as research method. In M. Leininger (Ed.), *Qualitative research methods in nursing* (pp. 73–80). Orlando, FL: Grune & Stratton.

Gaut, D. A (1986). Evaluating caring competencies in nursing practice. *Topics in Clinical Nursing, 8*(2), 77–83.

Gustafson, W. (1984). Motivational and historical aspects of care and nursing. In M. Leininger (Ed.), *Care: The essence of nursing and health* (pp. 61–73). Detroit, MI: Wayne State University Press.

Guthrie, B. (1981). The interrelatedness of the caring patterns in black children and caring process within black families. In M. Leininger (Ed.), *Caring: An essential human need* (pp. 103–107). Detroit, MI: Wayne State University Press.

Halldorsdottir, S. (1989). The essential structure of a caring and an uncaring encounter with a teacher: The nursing student's perspective. In M. Leininger & J. Watson (Eds.), *The caring imperative in education.* New York: National League for Nursing.

Halldorsdottir, S. (1991). Five basic modes of being with another. In D. Gaut & M. Leininger (Eds.), *Caring: The compassionate healer* (pp. 37–50). New York: National League for Nursing.

Kaplan, A. (1964). *The conduct of inquiry.* PA: Chandler Publishing.

Kleppe, H. (1987). Background and development of caring research in Norway. *Scandinavian Journal of Caring Sciences, 1*(3–4), 95–98.

Knowlden, V. (1988). Nurse caring as constructed knowledge. In R. Neil & R. Watts (Eds.), *Caring and nursing: Explorations in the feminist perspective* (pp. 318–339). New York: National League for Nursing.

Larson, P. (1984). Important nurse caring behaviors perceived by patients with cancer. *Oncology Nurse Forum, 11*(6), 46–50.

Larson, P. (1986). Cancer nurses' perceptions of caring. *Cancer Nursing, 9*(2), 86–91.

Leininger, M. (1978). *Transcultural nursing: Concepts, theories, and practices.* New York: Wiley.

Introduction

Leininger, M. (1981). Some philosophical, historical and taxonomic aspects of nursing and caring in American culture. In M. Leininger (Ed.), *Caring: An essential human need* (pp. 133–143). Detroit, MI: Wayne State University Press.

Leininger, M. (1991). *Culture care diversity and universality: A theory for nursing.* New York: National League for Nursing.

MacDonald, M. (1984). Caring: The central construct for an Associate Degree Nursing curriculum. In M. Leininger (Ed.), *Care: The essence of nursing and health* (pp. 233–248). Detroit, MI: Wayne State University Press.

Morse, J., Bottoroff, J., Neander, W., & Solberg, S. (1991). Comparative analysis of conceptualizations and theories of caring. *Image: The Journal of Nursing Scholarship, 23*(2), 119)–126.

Nyberg, J. (1989). The element of caring in nursing administration. *Nursing Administration Quarterly, 13*(3), 9–16.

Ray, M. (1981). A philosophical analysis of caring within nursing. In M. Leininger (Ed.), *Caring: An essential human need* (pp. 25–36). Detroit, MI: Wayne State University Press.

Ray M. (1984). The development of a classification system of institutional caring. In M. Leininger (Ed.), *Care: The essence of nursing and health* (pp. 95–112). Detroit, MI: Wayne State University Press.

Ray, M. (1985). A philosophical method to study nursing phenomena. In M. Leininger (Ed.), *Qualitative research methods in nursing* (pp. 81–92). Orlando, FL: Grune & Stratton.

Ray, M. (1989). The theory of bureaucratic caring for nursing practice in the organizational culture. *Nursing Administration Quarterly, 13*(2), 31–42.

Riemen, D. (1986A). Noncaring and caring in the clinical setting: Patients' descriptions. *Topics in Clinical Nursing, 8*(2), 30–36.

Riemen, D. (1986B). The essential structure of a caring interaction: Doing phenomenology. In Munhall & Oiler (Eds.), *Nursing research: A qualitative perspective* (pp. 85–108). Norwalk, CT: Appleton-Century-Crofts.

Roach, M. S. (1987). *The human act of caring: A blueprint for the health professions.* Ottawa: The Canadian Hospital Association Press.

Roach, M. S. (1992). *The human act of caring: A blueprint for the health professions (rev. ed.).* Ottawa: The Canadian Hospital Association Press.

Sherwood, G. (1991). Expressions of nurses' caring: The role of the compassionate healer. In D. Gaut & M. Leininger (Eds.) *Caring: The compassionate healer* (pp. 79–88). New York: National League for Nursing.

Smerke, J. (1989). *Interdisciplinary guide to the literature for human caring.* New York: National League for Nursing.

Swanson-Kauffman, (1986). A combined qualitative methodology for nursing research. *Advances in Nursing Science, 8*(3), 58–69.

Valentine, K. (1988). Advancing care and ethics in health management: An evaluation strategy. In M. Leininger (Ed.), *Care: Discovery and uses in clinical and community nursing* (pp. 151–167). Detroit, MI: Wayne State University Press.

Valentine, K. (1989). Caring is more than kindness: Modeling its complexities. *Journal of Nursing Administration, 19*(11), 28–34.

Valentine, K. (1991). Nurse–Patient caring: Challenging our conventional wisdom. In D. Gaut & M. Leininger (Eds.) *Caring: The compassionate healer* (pp. 99–113). New York: National League for Nursing.

Wang, J. (1984). Caretaker–child interaction observed in two Appalachian clinics. In M. Leininger (Ed.), *Care: The essence of nursing and health* (pp. 195–215). Detroit, MI: Wayne State University Press.

Watson, J. (1979). *Nursing: The philosophy and science of caring.* Boston: Little, Brown.

Watson, J. (1985A). *Nursing: Human science and human care. A theory of nursing.* Norwalk, CT: Appleton-Century-Crofts.

Introduction

Watson, J. (1985B). Reflections on different methodologies for the future of nursing. In M. Leininger (Ed.), *Qualitative research methods in nursing* (pp. 343–349). Orlando, FL: Grune & Stratton.

Watson J., Burckhardt, C., Brown, L., Bloch, D., & Hester, N. (1979). A model of caring: An alternative health care model for nursing practice and research. In *American Nurses' Association Clinical and Scientific Sessions.* Kansas City: American Nurses' Association Press.

Wenger, A. F. (1985). Learning to do a miniethnonursing research study. In M. Leininger (Ed.), *Qualitative research methods in nursing* (pp. 283–316).

Wenger, A. F. and Wenger, M. (1988). Community and family care patterns of the Old Order Amish. In M. Leininger (Ed.), *Care: Discovery and uses in clinical and community nursing* (pp. 39–54). Detroit, MI: Wayne State University Press.

Wesorick, B. (1990). *Standards of nursing care: A model for clinical practice.* Philadelphia: Lippincott.

Wesorick, B. (1991). Creating an environment in the hospital setting that supports caring via a clinical practice model. In D. Gaut & M. Leininger (Eds.), *Caring: The compassionate healer.* New York: National League for Nursing.

Whitehead, A. N. (1967). *Science and the modern world.* New York: Free Press.

Wolf, Z. 1986). The caring concept and nurse identified caring behaviors. *Topics in Clinical Nursing, 8*(2), 84–93.

ACKNOWLEDGEMENTS

*T*he authors gratefully acknowledge past and present faculty and students of the College of Nursing at Florida Atlantic University whose sharing through dialogue has contributed to the evolution of ideas over the past 12 years. We are particularly grateful to the faculty for taking the risks necessary to advance a program of study grounded in the discipline with caring as the focal point. Through supporting each other as colleagues, we were able to suspend our traditional pasts in order to study and teach the discipline with a new lens.

We also are indebted to students and colleagues whose questions, stories, and expressions of nursing fostered clarity in our understanding of the ontology of nursing. A special thank you goes to the following colleagues whose stories are re-presented in this book: Gayle Maxwell, Daniel Little, Sheila Carr, Patricia Kronk, Lorraine Wheeler, and Michele Stobie.

To the many scholars in the discipline whose works reflect a commitment to the development of nursing knowledge related to caring in nursing, and especially to the members of the International Association of Human Caring, we thank you. We extend a special thanks to Marilyn Parker and Terri Touhy for their unending devotion and commitment to nursing and for the blessing of their friendship.

We acknowledge Shawn Pennell who designed the image of the dance of caring persons described in this book. Sally Barhydt of the National League for Nursing offered understanding and thoughtful input in the early stages of this process and we thank her for her invaluable support. Thanks also to Allan Graubard of the League for his recognition of the meaning of our work, and for his careful attention in seeing this manuscript through to publication.

We would like to recognize all persons we have been privileged to nurse. Through the experience and study of these nursing situations, the knowledge of the discipline unfolds.

Last, we extend gratitude to our families for living caring with us and supporting our many professional endeavors.

1

FOUNDATIONS OF NURSING AS CARING

*I*n this chapter we present the fundamental ideas related to person as caring and nursing as a discipline and profession that serve as the perspectival grounding for the theory Nursing as Caring. We intend to offer our perspective of these ideas as influenced by the works of various scholars so that the grounding for Nursing as Caring will be understood. We do not intend to offer a novel perspective of the notion of person, a new generic understanding of caring, nor of discipline and profession, but to communicate some of the ideas basic to Nursing as Caring.

Major assumptions underlying Nursing as Caring include:

- persons are caring by virtue of their humanness
- persons are caring, moment to moment
- persons are whole or complete in the moment
- personhood is a process of living grounded in caring
- personhood is enhanced through participating in nurturing relationships with caring others
- nursing is both a discipline and profession.

PERSPECTIVE OF PERSONS AS CARING

Throughout this book the basic premise presides: *all persons are caring.* Caring is an essential feature and expression of being human. The belief that all persons, by virtue of their humanness, are caring establishes the ontological and ethical ground on which this theory is built. Persons as caring is a value which underlies each of the major concepts of Nursing as Caring and is an essential idea for understanding this theory and its implications. Being *person* means living caring, and it is through caring that our "being" and all possibilities are known to the fullest. Elaboration on the meaning of this perspective will provide a necessary backdrop for understanding ideas in subsequent chapters.

Caring is a process. Each person, throughout his or her life, grows in the capacity to express caring. Said another way, each person grows in their competency to express self as caring person. Because of our belief that each person is caring and grows in caring throughout life, we will not focus on behaviors considered noncaring in this book. Our assumption that all persons are caring does not require that every act of a person is necessarily caring. There are many experiences of life that teach us that not every act of a person is caring. These acts are obviously not expressions of self as caring person and may well be labelled noncaring. Developing the fullest potential for expressing caring is an ideal. Notwithstanding the abstract context of this ideal, it is *knowing* the person as living caring and growing in caring that is central to our effort in this book. Therefore, even though an act or acts may be interpreted as noncaring, the person remains caring.

While this assumption does not require that every act be understood as an expression of caring, the assumption that all persons are caring does require an acceptance that fundamentally, potentially, and actually each person is caring. Although persons are innately caring, actualization of the potential to express caring varies in the moment and develops over time. Thus, caring is lived moment to moment and is constantly unfolding. The development of competency in caring occurs over a lifetime. Throughout life we come to understand what it means to be a caring person, to live caring, and to nurture each other as caring.

Roach and Mayeroff provide some explanation as to what caring involves. Roach in her works (1984, 1987, 1992) has asserted that caring is the "human mode of being" (1992, p. ix).

As such, it entails the capacity to care, the calling forth of this ability in ourselves and others, responding to something or someone that matters and finally actualizing the ability to care (1992, p. 47). Since caring is a characteristic of being human, it cannot be attributed as a manifestation of any single discipline. These beliefs have directly influenced our assumption that all persons are caring. Mayeroff, a philosopher, in his 1971 book, *On Caring,* discusses caring as an end in itself, an ideal, and not merely a means to some future end. Within the context of caring as process, Roach (1992, 1984) says that caring entails the human capacity to care, the calling forth of this ability in ourselves and others, the responsivity to something or someone that matters, and the actualizing of the power to care. Even though our human nature is to be caring, the full expression of this varies with the lived experience of being human. The process of bringing forth this capability can be nurtured through concern and respect for person as person.

Mayeroff suggests that caring "is not to be confused with such meanings as wishing well, liking, comforting, and maintaining . . . it is not an isolated feeling or a momentary relationship" (p. 1). He describes caring as helping the other grow. In relationships lived through caring, changes in the one who cares and the one cared for are evident.

Mayeroff tells us how caring provides meaning and order:

> In the context of a man's life, caring has a way of ordering his other values and activities around it. When this advising is comprehensive, because of the inclusiveness of his caring, there is a basic stability in his life; he is "in place" in the world instead of being out of place, or merely drifting on endlessly seeking his place. Through caring for certain others, by serving them through caring a man lives the meaning of his own life. In the sense in which a man can ever be said to be at home in the world, he is at home not through dominating, or explaining, or appreciating, but through caring and being cared for (1971, p. 2).

Mayeroff expressed ideas about the meaning of being a caring person when he referred to trust as "being entrusted with the care of another" (p. 7). He spoke of both "being with" the other (p. 43) and "being for" (p. 42) the other, experiencing the other as an extension of self and at the same time "something separate from me that I respect in its own right" (p. 2). To be a caring person means to "live the meaning of my own life" (p. 72), having a sense of stability and basic certainty that allows an openness and accessibility, experiencing belonging, living congruence between beliefs and behavior, and expressing a clarity of values that enables living a simplified rather than a cluttered life.

Watson, a nursing theorist and philosopher, offers insight into caring. In her theory of Human Care, she examines caring as an intersubjective human process expressing respect for the mystery of being-in-the-world, reflected in the three spheres of mind-body-soul. Human care transactions based on reciprocity allow for an unique and authentic quality of presence in the world of the other. In a related vein, Parse (1981) defines the ontology of caring as "risking being with someone toward a moment of joy." Through being with another, connectedness occurs and moments of joy are experienced by both.

If the ontological basis for being is that all persons are caring and that by our humanness caring *is,* then I accept that I am a caring person. This belief that all persons are caring, however, entails a *commitment* to know self and other as caring person. According to Trigg (1973), commitment "presupposes certain beliefs and also involves a personal dedication to the actions implied by them" (p. 44). Mayeroff (1971) speaks of this dedication as devotion and states "devotion is essential to caring . . . when devotion breaks down, caring breaks down" (p. 8). Mayeroff also states that "obligations that derive from devotion are a constituent element in caring" (p. 9). Moral obligations arise from our commitments; therefore, when I make a commitment to caring as a way of being, I have become morally obligated. The quality of the moral commitment is a measure of being "in place" in the world. Gadow (1980) asserts that caring represents the moral ideal of nursing wherein the human dignity of the patient and nurse is recognized and enhanced.

As individuals we are continually in the process of developing expressions of ourselves as caring persons. The flow of life experiences provides ongoing opportunities for knowing self as caring person. As we learn to live fully each of these experiences, it becomes easier to allow self and others the space and time to develop innate caring capabilities and authentic being. The awareness of self as caring person calls to consciousness the belief that caring is lived by each person moment to moment and directs the "oughts" of actions. When decisions are made from this perspective, the emerging question consistently is, "How ought I act as caring person?"

How one is with others is influenced by the degree of authentic awareness of self as caring person. Caring for self as person requires experiencing self as other and yet being one with self, valuing self as special and unique, and having the courage, humility, and trust to honestly know self. It takes courage to let go of the present so that it may be transcended and new meaning be discovered. Letting go, of course, implies a freeing of oneself from present constraints so that we may see and be in new ways. One who cares is genuinely humble in being ready and willing to know more about self and others. Such humility involves the realization that learning is continuous and the recognition that each experience is new and unique. As my commitment to persons as caring moves into the future, I must choose again and again to ratify it or not. This commitment remains binding and choices are made based on devotion to this commitment.

Personhood is the process of living grounded in caring. Personhood implies living out who we are, demonstrating congruence between beliefs and behaviors, and living the meaning of one's life. As a process, personhood acknowledges the person as having continuous potential for further tapping the current of caring. Therefore, as person we are constantly living caring and unfolding possibilities for self as caring person in each moment. Personhood is being authentic, being who I am as caring person in the moment. This process is enhanced through participation in nurturing relationships with others.

The nature of relationships is transformed through caring. All relations between and among persons carry with them mutual expectations. Caring is living in the context of relational responsibilities. A relationship experienced through caring holds at its heart the importance of person-as-person. Being in the world also mandates participating in human relationships that require responsibility—responsibility to self and other. To the extent that these relationships are shaped through caring, they are consistent with the obligations entailed in relational responsibility, and the "person-al" (person-to-person) relationships. When being with self and others is approached from a desire to know person as living caring, the human potential for actualizing caring directs the moment.

All relationships are opportunities to draw forth caring possibilities, opportunities to reinforce the beauty of person-as-person. Through knowing self as caring person, I am able to be authentic to self and with others. I am able to see from the inside what others see from the outside. Feelings, attitudes, and actions lived in the moment are matched by an inner genuine awareness. The more I am open to knowing and appreciating self and trying to understand the world of other, the greater the awareness of our interconnectedness as caring persons. Knowing of self frees one to truly *be with* other. How does one come to know self as caring person? Mayeroff's

(1971) caring ingredients are useful conceptual tools when one is struggling to know self and other as caring. These ingredients include: honesty, courage, hope, knowing (both knowing about and knowing directly), trust, honesty, humility, and alternating rhythm.

The idea of a hologram serves as a way of understanding self and other. Pribram (1985) offers us an interesting view on relationships in his discussion of hologram. He states that the uniqueness of a hologram is such that if a part (of the hologram) is broken, any part of it is capable of reconstructing the total image (p. 133). Using this idea, if the lens for "being" in relationships is holographic, then the beauty of the person will be retained. Through entering, experiencing, and appreciating the world of other, the nature of being human is more fully understood. The notion of person as whole or complete expresses an important value. As such, the respect for the total person—all that is in the moment—is communicated. Therefore, from a holographic perspective, it is impossible to focus on a part of a person without seeing the whole person reflected in the part. The wholeness (the fullness of being) is forever present. Perhaps in some context, the word *part* is incongruent with this notion that there is only wholeness. The term *aspect,* or *dimension,* may be a useful substitute.

The view of person as caring and complete is also intentional; it offers a lens for a way of being with another that prevents the segmenting of that other into component parts (e.g., mind, body, spirit). Here, valuing and respecting each person's beauty, worth, and uniqueness is lived as one seeks to understand fully the meaning of values, choices, and priority systems through which values are expressed. The inherent value that persons reflect and to which they respond is the wholeness of persons. The person is at all times whole. The idea of wholeness does not negate an appreciation of the complexity of being. However, from the perspective of the theory

Nursing as Caring, to encounter person as less than whole involves a failure to encounter person. Until our view is such that it includes the whole as complete person and not just a part, we can not fully know the person. Gadow's (1984) contrasting paradigms, empathic and philanthropic, are relevant to this understanding. The philanthropic paradigm enables relationship in which dignity is bestowed as a "gift from one who is whole to one who is not" (p. 68). Philanthropy marks the person as other than one like me. Gadow's empathic paradigm, on the other hand, "breaches objectivity" (p. 67) and expresses participating in the experience of another. In the empathic paradigm, the subjectivity of the other is "assumed to be as whole and valid as that of the caregiver" (p. 68). These paradigm descriptions facilitate our knowing how we are with others. Is the attitude expressed through nursing one of person as part or person as whole? How do these perspectives direct nursing practice?

Our understanding of person as caring centers on valuing and celebrating human wholeness, the human person as living and growing in caring, and active personal engagement with others. This perspective of what it means to be human is the foundation for understanding nursing as a human endeavor, a person-to-person service, a human social institution, and a human science.

CONCEPTION OF NURSING AS DISCIPLINE AND PROFESSION

In this work, our second major perspectival grounding involves a social conception of nursing as a discipline and a profession. Here, ideas such as *social contract* and *human science* are important to understanding the scope and significance of this new and developing general theory of Nursing as Caring. Since the theory evolved from a stance that nursing is both a discipline and a profession, a discussion of characteristics of both social structures lays crucial groundwork.

The discipline of nursing and the profession of nursing are inextricably bound and exquisitely interwoven aspects of the single unity of nursing. Each aspect illuminates particular duties, privileges, and realms of activity relevant to nursing as an entity. The discipline of nursing has its origins in the unique social call upon the world to which the practice of nursing is a response. The profession of nursing involves professing an understanding of both the social need from which the calls for nursing arise and the body of knowledge drawn upon in creating the nursing response.

In this regard, the nature of nursing takes on new dimensions as the domain of nursing knowledge gains clear articulation. As mentioned, our work is predicated on the understanding that nursing is a discipline—a way of knowing, being, valuing, and living. This conception transcends the somewhat artificial divisions between science, ethic, and art as distinct entities, and unifies nursing as a practiced discipline. Our understanding of nursing as a discipline has been enriched by our use of the work of Phenix (1964), King and Brownell (1976), and the Nursing Development Conference Group (1979). Further, building on Carper's (1978) application of Phenix to nursing knowledge, it has become clear that addressing nursing as science, ethic or art, or partitioning nursing into those dimensions, is not adequate for the development of nursing as a unique discipline. Instead, we envision nursing as a unity of knowledge within a larger unity. Knowing nursing, therefore means knowing in the realms of personal, ethical, empirical, and aesthetic—all at once. When that which is known as nursing is known solely as science, or as art, the knowing is not adequate to the requirements of nursing practice, nursing education, or nursing scholarship.

King and Brownell (1976) have ably described the essential characteristics that define disciplines. In this regard, the discipline of nursing is represented by a community of scholars dedicated to developing a particular field of knowledge representing a unique view of humankind and human endeavor. Of course, the domain of any discipline, including nursing, is that which its members assert. The domain embodies the valuative and affective stance taken, and implies acceptance of responsibility for the discourse of the discipline. In its most fundamental sense then, a discipline is understood as a pathway of knowing and being in the world. We do not intend that our view of nursing as a discipline denigrate efforts of the past or present. Rather, we believe our view enables the development of nursing as a discipline of constant discovery and new knowing.

Like disciplines, professions have unique characteristics, as defined by Flexner. Flexner (1910) initially identified as the most basic characteristic of a profession that it addresses an unique and urgent social need through techniques derived from a tested knowledge base. Professions have their historical roots in those human services that people provided for each other within existing social institutions (e.g., tribe, family, or community). Thus, each profession, including nursing, has its origins in everyday human situations and the everyday contributions people make to the welfare of others. Flexner's founding condition for the designation *profession* is reiterated in the American Nursing Association's 1980 Social Policy Statement, in which the idea of a social contract is addressed.

Nursing: A Social Policy Statement was intended to provide nurses with a fresh perspective on practice while providing society with a view of nursing for the 1980s. The overall intent of this document was to call to consciousness the linkages between the profession and society. While the "Social Policy Statement" is considered by many (see, for example, Rodgers, 1991; Packard & Polifroni, 1991; Allen 1987; White, 1984) to be outdated, we find the concept of the social contract to be useful when studying the relationship of nurse to nursed. As the foundation for professions, the social contract, while understood to be an "hypothetical ideal" (Silva, 1983, p. 150), is also an expression of a people recognizing (1) the presence of a basic need and (2) the existence of greater knowledge and skill available to meet that need than can be readily exercised by each member of the society. Society at large then calls for commitment by a segment of society to the acquisition and use of this knowledge and skill for the good of all. Social goods are promised in return for this commitment.

Today, the profession of nursing is moving from a social contract relationship toward a covenantal relationship between the nurse and nursed. While the social contract implies an impersonal, legalistic stance, the covenantal relationship emphasizes personal engagement and ever present freedom to choose commitments. Cooper (1988), for example, discusses her ideas on the relevance of covenantal relationships for nursing ethics. She states that "the promissory nature of the covenant is contained in the willingness of individuals to enter a covenantal relationship" (p. 51) and it is within this context that obligations arise. As caring persons, we "see" relationship (covenant) and honor the bond between self and other. The ultimate knowledge gained from this perspective is that we are related to one another (and to the universe) and that harmony (brotherhood and sisterhood) is present as we live out caring relationships.

Concepts of discipline and profession have been dismissed by critical theorists as oppressive, anachronistic, and paternalistic (Allen, 1985; Rodgers, 1991). In our study however, as we have explored essential meanings of these concepts, we have found that they express fundamental values congruent with cherished nursing values. Although we can agree with critical theorists that discipline and profession have been misused, perhaps too frequently, as tools of social elitism and oppression, this misuse remains inappropriate because it violates the covenantal nature of discipline and profession.

The discipline of nursing attends to the discovery, creation, structuring, testing, and refinement of knowledge needed for the practice of nursing. Concomitantly, the profession of nursing attends to the use of that knowledge in response to specific human needs. Certainly, the basic values communicated in the concepts of discipline and profession are resonate with fundamental nursing values and contribute to a fuller understanding of nursing as caring. Included among those shared values are commitment to something that matters, sense of persons being connected in oneness; expression of human imagination and creativity, realization of the unity of knowing with possibilities unfolding, and expression of choice and responsibility.

We have deliberately used the term *general theory of nursing* to characterize our work. The concept of a general theory is particularly useful in the context of levels of theory. Other authors have addressed what they see as three levels of nursing theory: general or grand, mid-range, and practice (Walker & Avant, 1988; Fawcett, 1989; Chinn & Jacobs, 1987; Nursing Development Conference Group, 1979). What we intend by the use of the term *general theory* is similar to "conceptual framework," "conceptual model," or "paradigm." That is, a general theory is a framework for understanding any and all instances of nursing, and may be used to describe or to project any given situation of nursing. It is a system of values ordered specifically to reflect a philosophy of nursing to guide knowledge generation and to inform practice.

The statement of focus of any general nursing theory offers an explicit expression of the social need that calls for and justifies the professional service of nursing. In addition, the statement of focus expresses the domain of a discipline as well as the intent of the profession, and thus directs the development of the requisite nursing knowledge. Activity to develop and use nursing knowledge has its ethical ground in the idea of the covenantal relationship as expressed in the specific focus of the profession. Fundamental values inherent in the discipline and profession of nursing derive from an understanding of the focus of nursing.

The conception of nursing that we have used in this book views nursing science as a form of human science. Nursing as caring focuses on the knowledge needed to understand the fullness of what it means to be human and on the methods to verify this knowledge. For this reason, we have not accepted the traditional notion of theory which relies on the "received" view of science, and depends on measurement as the ultimate tool for legitimate knowledge development. The human science of nursing requires the use of all ways of knowing.

Carper's (1978) fundamental patterns of knowing in nursing are useful conceptual tools for expanding our view of nursing science as human science here. These patterns provide an organizing framework for asking epistemological questions of caring in nursing. To experience knowing the whole of a nursing situation with caring as the central focus, each of these patterns comes into play. Personal knowing focuses on knowing and encountering self and other intuitively, the empirical pathway addresses the senses, ethical knowing focuses on moral knowing of what "ought to be" in nursing situations, and esthetic knowing involves the appreciating and creating that integrates all patterns of knowing in relation to a particular situation. Through the richness of the knowledge gleaned, the nurse as artist creates the caring moment (Boykin & Schoenhofer, 1990).

Nursing, as we have come to understand our discipline, is not a normative science that stands outside a situation to evaluate current observations against empirically derived and tested normative standards. Nursing as a human science takes its value from the knowledge created within the shared lived experience of the unique nursing situation. Although empirical facts and norms do play a role in nursing knowledge, we must remember that that role is not one of unmediated application. Knowledge of nursing comes from within the situation. The nurse reaches out into a body of normative information, transforming that information as understanding is created from within the situation. The same can be said for personal and ethical knowing. Each serves as a pathway for transforming knowledge in the creation of esthetic knowing within the nursing situation. The view we have taken unifies previously dichotomized notions of nursing as science and nursing as art and requires a new understanding of science.

Nursing as caring reflects an appreciation of persons in the fullness of personhood within the context of the nursing situation. This view transcends perspectives adopted in an earlier period of nursing science philosophy. Examples of the earlier view include the notions of basic versus applied science, and metaphysics versus theory. The idea of a basic science of nursing disconnects nursing from its very ground of ethical value. Without a grounding in praxis, the content and activity of nursing science becomes amoral and meaningless. Similarly, this view transcends an earlier view of nursing theory that treated the unitary phenomenon of nursing as being composed of concepts that could be studied independently or as "independent and dependent variables." Nursing as caring resists fragmentation of the unitary phenomenon of our discipline. In subsequent chapters, we will more fully explore the implications of this view of nursing as a human science discipline and profession.

REFERENCES

Allen, D. G. (1985). Nursing research and social control: Alternative models of science that emphasize understanding and emancipation. *Image, 17*(2), 59–64.

Allen, D. G. (1987). The social policy statement; A reappraisal. *Advances in Nursing Science, 10*(1), 39–48.

American Nurses Association. (1980). *Nursing: A social policy statement.* Kansas City: American Nurses Association.

Boykin, A., & Schoenhofer, S. (1990). Caring in nursing: Analysis of extant theory. *Nursing Science Quarterly, 4,* 149–155.

Carper, B. (1978). Fundamental patterns of knowing in nursing. *Advances in Nursing Science, 1,* 13–24.

Chinn, P., & Jacobs, M. (1987). *Theory and nursing.* St. Louis: Mosby.

Cooper, M. C. (1988). Covenantal relationships: Grounding for the nursing ethic. *Advances in Nursing Science, 10*(4), 48–59.

Fawcett, T. (1989). *Analysis and evaluation of conceptual models of nursing.* Philadelphia: F. A. Davis.

Flexner, A. (1910). *Medical education in the United States and Canada.* New York: Carnegie Foundation.

Gadow, S. (1980). Existential advocacy: Philosophical foundations of nursing. In S. Spicker & Gadow, S., (Eds.), *Nursing: Images and Ideals.* New York: Springer, pp. 79–101.

Gadow, S. (1984). Touch and technology: Two paradigms of patient care. *Journal of Religion and Health, 23,* 63–69.

King, A., & Brownell, J. (1976). *The curriculum and the disciplines of knowledge.* Huntington, NY: Robert E. Krieger Publishing Co.

Mayeroff, M. (1971). *On caring.* New York: Harper & Row.

Nursing Development Conference Group (1979). *Concept formalization in nursing: Process and product.* Boston: Little, Brown.

Packard, S. A., & Polifroni, E. C. (1991). The dilemma of nursing science: Current quandaries and lack of direction. *Nursing Science Quarterly, 4*(1), 7–13.

Parse, R. (1981). Caring from a human science perspective. In M. Leininger (Ed.). *Caring: An essential human need.* Thorofare, NJ: Slack. (Reissued by Wayne State University Press, Detroit, 1988).

Phenix, P. (1964). *Realms of meaning.* New York: McGraw-Hill.

Pribram, K. H. (1971). *Languages of the brain: Experimental paradoxes and principles in neuropsychology.* Englewood Cliffs, NJ: Prentice-Hall.

Roach, S. (1984). *Caring: The human mode of being, implications for nursing.* Toronto: Faculty of Nursing, University of Toronto.

Roach, S. (1987). *The human act of caring.* Ottawa: Canadian Hospital Association.

Roach, S. (1992 Revised). *The human act of caring.* Ottawa: Canadian Hospital Association.

Rodgers, B. L. (1991). Deconstructing the dogma in nursing knowledge and practice. *Image, 23*(2), 177–181.

Silva, M. C. (1983). The American Nurses' Association position statement on nursing and social policy: Philosophical and ethical dimensions. *Journal of Advanced Nursing, 8*(2), 147–151.

Tillich, P. (1952). *The courage to be.* New Haven: Yale University Press.

Trigg, R. (1973). *Reason and commitment.* London: Cambridge University Press.

Walker, L., & Avant, K. (1988). *Strategies for theory construction in nursing.* Norwalk, CT: Appleton & Lange.

Watson, J. (1988; 1985). *Nursing: Human science and human care, a theory of nursing.* Norwalk, CT: Appleton-Century-Crofts.

White, C. M. (1984). A critique of the ANA Social Policy Statement . . . population and environment focused nursing. *Nursing Outlook, 32*(6), 328–331.

2

NURSING AS CARING

*I*n Chapter 2, we will present the general theory of Nursing as Caring. Here, the unique focus of nursing is posited as *nurturing persons living caring and growing in caring.* While we will discuss the meaning of that statement of focus in general terms, we will also describe specific concepts inherent in this focus in the context of the general theory.

If you recall, in Chapter 1 we discussed the several major assumptions that ground the theory of Nursing as Caring:

- Persons are caring by virtue of their humanness
- Persons are whole or complete in the moment
- Persons live caring, moment to moment
- Personhood is a process of living grounded in caring
- Personhood is enhanced through participating in nurturing relationships with caring others
- Nursing is both a discipline and profession

In this and succeeding chapters, we will develop the nursing implications of these assumptions.

All persons are caring. This is the fundamental view that grounds the focus of nursing as a discipline and a profession. The unique perspective offered by the theory of Nursing as Caring builds on that view by recognizing personhood as a process of living grounded in caring. This is meant to imply that the fullness of being human is expressed as one lives caring uniquely day to day. The process of living grounded in caring is enhanced through participation in nurturing relationships with caring others, particularly in nursing relationships.

Within the theoretical perspective given herein, a further major assumption appears: persons are viewed as already complete and continuously growing in completeness, fully caring and unfolding caring possibilities moment-to-moment. Such a view assumes that caring is being lived by each of us, moment to moment. Expressions of self as caring person are complete in the moment as caring possibilities unfold; thus, notwithstanding other life contingencies, one continues to grow in caring competency, in fully expressing self as caring person. To say that one is fully caring in the moment also involves a recognition of the uniqueness of person with each moment presenting new possibilities to know self as caring person. The notion of "in the moment" reflects the idea that competency in knowing self as caring and as living caring grows throughout life. Being complete in the moment also signifies something more: there is no insufficiency, no brokenness, or absence of something. As a result, nursing activities are not directed toward *healing* in the sense of making whole; from our perspective, wholeness is present and unfolding. There is no lack, failure, or inadequacy which is to be corrected through nursing—persons are whole, complete, and caring.

The theory of Nursing as Caring, then, is based on an understanding that the focus of nursing, both as a discipline and as a profession, involves the nurturing of persons living caring and growing in caring. In this statement of focus, we recognize the unique human need to which nursing is the response as a desire to be recognized as caring person and to be supported in caring.

This focus also requires that the nurse know the person seeking nursing as caring person and that the nursing actions be directed toward nurturing the nursed in their living caring and growing in caring. We will briefly discuss this theory in general terms here and more fully illuminate it in subsequent chapters on nursing practice (Chapter 4), education (Chapter 5), and scholarship (Chapter 6). We will address administration of nursing services and of nursing education programs in Chapters 4 and 5, respectively.

Nurturing persons living caring and growing in caring at first glance appears broad and abstract. In some ways, the focus is broad in that it applies to nursing situations in a wide variety of practice settings. On the other hand, it takes on specific and practical meaning in the context of individual nursing situations as the nurse attempts to know the nursed as caring person and focuses on nurturing that person as he or she lives and grows in caring.

When approaching a situation from this perspective, we understand each person as fundamentally caring, living caring in his or her everyday life. Forms of expressing one's unique ways of living caring are limited only by the imagination. Recognizing unique personal ways of living caring also requires an ethical commitment and knowledge of caring. In our everyday lives, failures to express caring are readily recognized. The ability to articulate instances of noncaring does not seem to take any particular skill. When nursing is called for, however, it is necessary that nurses have the commitment, knowledge, and skill to discover the individual unique caring person to be nursed. For example, the nurse may encounter one who may be described as despairing. Relating to that person as helpless recalls Gadow's (1984) characterization of the philanthropic paradigm which assumes "sufficiency and independence on one side and needy dependence on the other" (p. 68). The relationship grounded in nursing as caring would enable the nurse to connect with the hope that underlies an expression of despair or hopelessness. Personal expressions such as despair, or fear, or anger, for example, are neither ignored nor discounted. Rather, they are understood as the caring value which is in some way present. An honest expression of fear or anger, for example, is also an expression of vulnerability, which expresses courage and humility. We reiterate that our approach is grounded in the fundamental assumption that all persons are caring and the commitment which arises from this basic value position.

It is this understanding of person as caring that directs professional nursing decision making and action from the point of view of our Nursing as Caring theory. The nurse enters into the world of the other person with the intention of knowing the other as caring person. It is in knowing the other in their "living caring and growing in caring" that calls for nursing are heard. Of equal importance is our coming to know *how* the other is living caring in the situation and expressing aspirations for growing in caring. The call for nursing is a call for acknowledgement and affirmation of the person living caring in specific ways in this immediate situation. The call for nursing says "know me as caring person now and affirm me." The call for nursing evokes specific caring responses to sustain and enhance the other as they live caring and grow in caring in the situation of concern. This caring nurturance is what we call the nursing response.

NURSING SITUATION

The *nursing situation* is a key concept in the theory of Nursing as Caring. Thus, we understand *nursing situation as a shared lived experience in which the caring between nurse and nursed enhances personhood*. The nursing situation is the locus of all that is known and done in nursing. It is in this context that nursing lives. The content and structure of nursing knowledge are known through the study of the nursing situation. The content of nursing knowledge is generated, developed, conserved, and known through the lived experience of the nursing situation. Nursing situation as a construct is constituted in the mind of the nurse when the nurse conceptualizes or prepares

Nursing as Caring

to conceptualize a call for nursing. In other words, when a nurse engages in any situation from a nursing focus, a nursing situation is constituted.

In the Scandanavian countries, for instance, all the helping disciplines are called *caring sciences*. Professions such as medicine, social work, clinical psychology, and pastoral counseling have a caring function; however, caring per se is not their focus. Rather, the focus of each of these professions addresses particular forms of caring or caring in particular ranges of life situations. In nursing situations, the nurse focuses on nurturing persons as they live and grow in caring. While caring is not unique to nursing, it is uniquely expressed in nursing. The uniqueness of caring in nursing lies in the intention expressed by the statement of focus. As an expression of nursing, *caring is the intentional and authentic presence of the nurse with another who is recognized as person living caring and growing in caring. Here, the nurse endeavors to come to know the other as caring person and seeks to understand how that person might be supported, sustained, and strengthened in their unique process of living caring and growing in caring.* Again, each person in interaction in the nursing situation is known as caring. Each person grows in caring through interconnectedness with other.

Calls for nursing are calls for nurturance through personal expressions of caring, and originate within persons who are living caring in their lives and hold dreams and aspirations of growing in caring. Again, the nurse responds to the call of the caring person, not to some determination of an absence of caring. The contributions of each person in the nursing situation are also directed toward a common purpose, the nurturance of the person in their living and growing in caring.

In responding to the nursing call, the nurse brings an expert (expert in the sense of deliberately developed) knowledge of what it means to be human, to be caring, as a fully developed commitment to recognizing and nurturing caring in all situations. The nurse enters the other's world in order to know the person as caring. The nurse comes to know how caring is being lived in the moment, discovering unfolding possibilities for growing in caring. This knowing clarifies the nurse's understanding of the call and guides the nursing response. In this context, the general knowledge the nurse brings to the situation is transformed through an understanding of the uniqueness of that particular situation.

Every nursing situation is a lived experience involving at least two unique persons. Therefore, each nursing situation differs from any other. The reciprocal nature of the lived experience of the nursing situation requires a personal investment of both caring persons. The initial focus is on knowing persons as caring, both nurse and nursed. The process for knowing self and other as caring involves a constant and mutual unfolding. In order to know the other, the nurse must be willing to risk entering the other's world. For his or her part, the other person must be willing to allow the nurse to enter his or her world. For this to happen, the acceptance of trust and strength of courage needed by persons in the nursing situation can be awe-inspiring.

It is through the openness and willingness in the nursing situation that presence with other occurs. Presence develops as the nurse is willing to risk entering the world of the other and as the other invites the nurse into a special, intimate space. The encountering of the nurse and the nursed gives rise to a phenomenon we call *caring between,* within which personhood is nurtured. The nurse as caring person is fully present and gives the other time and space to grow. Through presence and intentionality, the nurse is able to know the other in his or her living and growing in caring. This personal knowing enables the nurse to respond to the unique call for nurturing personhood. Of course, responses to nursing calls are as varied as the calls themselves. All truly nursing responses are expressions of caring and are directed toward nurturing persons as they live and grow in caring in the situation.

In the situation, the nurse draws on personal, empirical, and ethical knowing to bring to life the artistry of nursing. When the nurse, as artist, creates unique approaches to care based on the dreams and goals of the one cared for, the moment comes alive with possibilities. Through the aesthetic, the nurse is free to know and express the beauty of the caring moment (Boykin & Schoenhofer, 1991). This full engagement within the nursing situation allows the nurse to truly experience nursing as caring, and to share that experience with the one nursed.

In Chapter 1, we noted that each profession arose from some everyday service given by one person to another. Nursing has long been associated with the idea of mothering, when mothering is understood as nurturing the personhood of another. The ideal mother (and father) recognizes the child as caring person, perfect in the moment and unfolding possibilities for becoming. The parent acknowledges and affirms the child as caring person and provides the caring environment that nurtures the child in living and growing in caring. The origins of nursing may well be found in the intimacy of parental caring. The roles of both parent and nurse permit and at times even expect that one be involved in the intimacy of the daily life of another. The parent is present in all situations to care for the child. Ideally, parents know the child as eminently worthwhile and caring, despite all the limitations and human frailties. As we recognized in Chapter 1, professions arise from the special needs of everyday situations, and nursing has perhaps emerged in relation to a type of caring that is synonymous with parenthood and friendship. The professional nurse, schooled in the discipline of nursing, brings expert knowledge of human caring to the nursing situation.

Nursing as Caring

In the early years of nursing model development, nursing scholars endeavored to articulate their discipline using the perspective of another discipline, for example, medicine, sociology, or psychology. One example of this endeavor is the Roy Adaptation Model, in which scientific assumptions reflect von Bertalanffy's general systems theory and Helson's adaptation level theory (Roy and Andrews, 1991, p. 5). Parson's theory of Social System Analysis is reflected in Johnson's Behavioral System Model for Nursing and Orem's Self Care Deficit Theory of Nursing (Meleis, 1985). A second trend involved declaring that the uniqueness of nursing was in the way in which it integrated and applied concepts from other disciplines. The emphasis in the 1960s on nursing model development came as an effort to articulate and structure the substance of nursing knowledge. This work was needed to enhance nursing education, previously based on rules of practice, and to provide a foundation for an emerging interest in nursing research. Nursing scholars engaged in model development as an expression of their commitment to the advancement of nursing as a discipline and profession, and we applaud their contributions. It is our view, however, that these early models, grounded in other disciplines, do not directly address the essence of nursing. The development of Nursing as Caring has benefited from these earlier efforts as well as from the work of more recent scholarship that posits caring as the central construct and essence (Leininger, 1988), and the moral ideal of Nursing (Watson, 1985).

The perspective of nursing presented here is notably different from most conceptual models and general theories in the field. The most radical difference becomes apparent in the form of the call for nursing. Most extant nursing theories, modelled after medicine and other professional fields, present the formal occasion for nursing as a problem, need, or deficit (e.g., Self-Care Deficit Theory [Orem, 1985], Adaptation

Nursing [Roy & Andrews, 1991], Behavioral System Model [Johnson, 1980], and Neuman Systems Model [Neuman, 1989]). Such theories then explain how nursing acts to right the wrong, meet the need, or eliminate or ameliorate the deficit.

The theory of Nursing as Caring proceeds from a frame of reference based on interconnectedness and collegiality rather than on esoteric knowledge, technical expertise, and disempowering hierarchies. In contrast, our emerging theory of nursing is based on an egalitarian model of helping that bears witness to and celebrates the human person in the fullness of his or her being, rather than on some less-than-whole condition of being.

REFERENCES

Boykin, A., & Schoenhofer, S. (1991). Story as link between nursing practice, ontology, epistemology. *Image, 23*, 245–248.

Gadow, S. (1984). Touch and technology: Two paradigms of patient care. *Journal of Religion and Health, 23*, 63–69.

Johnson, D. E. (1980). The behavioral system model of nursing. In J. Riehl & C. Roy (Eds.), *Conceptual models for nursing practice* (2nd ed.). New York: Appleton-Century-Crofts.

Leininger, M. M. (1988). Leininger's theory of nursing: Cultural care diversity and universality. *Nursing Science Quarterly, 1*, 152–160.

Meleis, A. (1985). *Theoretical nursing: Development & progress.* Philadelphia: J. B. Lippencott.

Neuman, B. (1989). *The Neumans systems model.* Norwalk, CT: Appleton & Lange.

Orem, D. E. (1985). *Nursing: Concepts of practice* (3rd ed.). New York: McGraw Hill.

Nursing as Caring

Roy, C., & Andrews, H. (1991). *The Roy Adaptation Model: The definitive statement.* Norwalk, CT: Appleton & Lange.

Watson, J. (1985). *Nursing: Human science and human care. A theory of nursing.* Norwalk, CT: Appleton-Century-Crofts.

3

NURSING SITUATION AS LOCUS OF NURSING

*T*he concept of nursing situation is central to every aspect of the theory of Nursing as Caring. We have claimed that all nursing knowledge resides within the nursing situation (Boykin & Schoenhofer, 1991). The nursing situation is both the repository of nursing knowledge and the context for knowing nursing. The nursing situation is known as a shared lived experience in which the caring between the nurse and the one nursed enhances personhood.

It is to the nursing situation that the nurse brings self as caring person. It is within the nursing situation that the nurse comes to know the other as caring person, expressing unique ways of living and growing in caring. And it is in the nursing situation that the nurse attends to calls for caring, creating caring responses that nurture personhood. It is within the nursing situation that the nurse comes to know nursing, in the fullness of aesthetic knowing.

The nursing situation comes into being when the nurse actualizes a personal and professional commitment to the belief that all persons are caring. It should be recognized that a nurse can engage in many activities in an occupational role that are not necessarily expressions of nursing. When a nurse practices nursing thoughtfully, that nurse is guided by his or her conception of nursing. The concept of nursing formalized in the Nursing as Caring theory is at the very heart of nursing, extending back into the unrecorded beginnings of nursing and forward into the future. Acknowledgement of caring as the core of nursing implies that any nurse, practicing nursing thoughtfully, is creating and living nursing situations because, whether explicit or tacit, the caring intent of nursing is present.

Remembering that the nursing situation is a construct held by the nurse, any interpersonal experience contains the potential to become a nursing situation. In the formal sense of professional nursing, the nursing situation develops when one person presents self in the role of offering the professional service of nursing and the other presents self in the role of seeking, wanting, or accepting nursing service.

The nurse intentionally enters the situation for the purpose of coming to know the other as caring person. The nurse is also allowing self to be known as caring person. Authentic presence, like most human capacities, is inherent and can be more fully developed through intention and deliberate effort. Authentic presence may be understood simply as one's intentionally being there with another in the fullness of one's personhood. Caring communicated through authentic presence is the initiating and sustaining medium of nursing within the nursing situation.

The nurse, with developed authentic presence and open to knowing the other as caring, begins to understand the other's call for nursing. A call for nursing is a call for specific forms of caring that acknowledge, affirm, and sustain the other as they strive to live caring uniquely. We must remember as well that calls for nursing originate within the unique relationship of the nursing situation. As the situation ensues, the call for nursing clarifies. The nurse comes to know the one nursed more and more deeply and to understand more fully the unique meaning of the person's caring ways and aspirations for growing in caring. It is in this understanding that the call for nursing is known as a specific situated expression of caring and a call for explicit caring response.

The nursing response of caring is also uniquely lived within each nursing situation. In the nursing situation, the call of the nursed is a personal "reaching out" to a hoped-for other. The nursed calls forth the nurse's personal caring response. While the range and scope of human caring expression can and must be studied, the caring response called forth in each nursing situation is created for that moment. The nurse responds to each call for nursing in a way that uniquely represents the fullness (wholeness) of the nurse. How I might respond to such a call would and should reflect my unique living of caring as person and nurse. Each response to a particular nursing situation would be slightly different and would portray the beauty of the nurse as person.

The nursing situation is a shared lived experience. The nurse joins in the life process of the person nursed and brings his or her life process to the relationship as well. In the nursing situation, there is caring between the participants. Further, the experience of the caring within the nursing situation enhances personhood, the process of living grounded in caring. Each of these components of the construct of the nursing situation raises questions for immediate and continuing discussion.

How can an unconscious patient be a participant in a nursing situation? Can "postmortem care" be considered nursing? How can the nurse know that the other is truly open to nursing—can the nurse impose self into the world of the other? What about an unrepentant child rapist or a person responsible for genocide, can we say that person is caring, and if not, can we nurse them? Does the nurse have to like the person being nursed? Does the nurse seek enhancement of personhood in the nursing situation? If so, might the goals of the nurse be imposed on the one nursed? If the nurse gains from the nursing situation, isn't that unprofessional?

In part, these legitimate questions raise larger issues about the uniqueness and scope of nursing as a discipline and professional service in society. Certainly the study of these questions adds clarity to the purpose of nursing actions. To nurse, situations in a general sense are transcended and transformed when they are conceptualized as nursing situations. From the perspective of the Nursing as Caring theory, the study of these questions would require that the nurse transcend social or other situational contexts and live out a commitment to nurture the person in the nursing situation as they live and grow in caring.

Persons with altered levels of consciousness, measured on normative scales developed for medical science purposes, can and do participate in nursing situations. Nurses committed to knowing the unconscious as caring person can and do describe their ways of expressing caring and aspirations for growing in caring. Nurses speak of the post-anesthesia patient as living hope in their struggle to emerge from the deadening effects of the anesthesia; as living honesty in fretful, fearful thrashing. Nurses help these persons sustain hope and extend honesty through their care. The profoundly mentally disabled child lives humility moment-to-moment and calls forth caring responses to validate and nurture that beautiful humility. Nurses speak of caring for their deceased patients as nursing those who have gone and are still in some way present. The nurse, connected in oneness with the one known and nursed, holds hope for the other as the other's expression of hopefulness lives on in the consciousness of the nurse. Thus, a sense of connectedness does not dissipate when physical presence ends, but remains an active part of the nurse's experience.

Nursing another is a service of caring, communicated through authentic presence. Nursing another means living out a commitment to knowing the other as caring person and responding to the caring other as someone of value (Boykin & Schoenhofer, 1990, 1991). In its fullest sense, nursing cannot be rendered impersonally, but must be offered in a spirit of being connected in oneness. "To care for" seems to require that the caregiver see oneself as caring person reflected in the other (Watson, 1987). The theoretical perspective of Nursing as Caring is grounded in the belief that caring is the human mode of being (Roach, 1984). When a person is judged by social standards to be deviant and even evil, however, it is difficult to summon caring. This points to the contribution nursing is called upon to make in society. When we speak of nursing's contribution here, we are invoking earlier discussions of discipline and profession. Each discipline and profession illuminates a special aspect of person—in effect, what it means to be human. The light that nursing shines on the world of person is knowledge of person as caring, so that the particular contribution of nursing is to illuminate the person as caring, living caring uniquely in situation and growing in caring. In nursing, practiced within the context of Nursing as Caring, the person is taken at face value as caring and never needs to prove him or herself as caring. The nurse, practicing within the context of Nursing as Caring, is skilled at recognizing and affirming caring in self and others.

Being caring, that is, living one's commitment to this value "important-in-itself" (Roach, 1984), fuels the nurse's growing in caring and enables the nurse in turn to nurture others in their living and growing in caring. The values and assumptions of nursing as caring can assist the nurse to engage fully in nursing situations with persons where caring is difficult to discover.

Nursing knowledge is discovered and tested in the ongoing nursing situations. Once experienced, nursing situations can be made available for living anew, with new discovery and testing. Aesthetic representation of nursing situations brings the lived experience into the realm of new experience. Thus, the knowledge of nursing can be made available for further study. Re-presentation of nursing situations can occur through the medium of nursing stories, poetry, painting, sculpture, and other art forms (Schoenhofer, 1989). Aesthetic re-presentation conserves the epistemic integrity of nursing while permitting full appreciation of the singularity of any one nursing situation (Boykin & Schoenhofer, 1991). Here, then, is one nurse's story of a shared lived experience in which the caring between nurse and the one nursed enhanced personhood. This story is offered as an example of nursing situation, re-presented as an open text, available for continuing participation by all who wish to enter into this shared lived experience of nursing. In fact, we invite the reader to enter into this nursing situation, which may then be used in classroom or conference settings to stimulate general or specific inquiry and dialogue.

Connections

One night as I listened to the change of shift report, I remember the strange feeling in the pit of my stomach when the evening nurse reviewed the lab tests on Tracy P. Tall, strawberry-blonde and freckle-faced, Tracy was struggling with the everyday problems of adolescence and fighting a losing battle against leukemia. Tracy rarely had visitors. As I talked with Tracy this night I felt resentment from her toward her mother, and I experienced a sense of urgency that her mother be with her. With Tracy's permission I called her mother and told her that Tracy needed her that night. I learned she was a single mother with two other small children, and that she lived several hours from the hospital. When she arrived at the hospital, distance and silence prevailed. With encouragement, the mother sat close to Tracy and I sat on the other side, stroking Tracy's arm. I left the room to make rounds and upon return found Mrs. P. still sitting on the edge of the bed fighting to stay awake. I gently asked Tracy if we could lie on the bed with her. She nodded. The three of us lay there for a period of time and I then left the room. Later, when I returned, I found Tracy wrapped in her mother's arms. Her mother's eyes met mine as she whispered "she's gone." And then, "please don't take her yet." I left the room and closed the door quietly behind me. It was just after

6 o'clock when I slipped back into the room just as the early morning light was coming through the window. "Mrs. P," I reached out and touched her arm. She raised her tear-streaked face to look at me. "It's time," I said and waited. When she was ready, I helped her off the bed and held her in my arms for a few moments. We cried together. "Thank you, nurse," she said as she looked into my eyes and pressed my hand between hers. Then she turned and walked away. The tears continued down my cheeks as I followed her to the door and watched her disappear down the hall.

Gayle Maxwell (1990)

This nursing situation is replete with possibilities for nurses, and others, to understand nursing as nurturing persons living caring and growing in caring. A dialogue ensues on the nursing situation that allows participants an opportunity to experience both resonance and uniqueness as personal and shared understandings emerge. As the reader enters into the text, the nursing situation is experienced anew, now within the presence of two nurses, not one. Through intentionally entering the situation, the second nurse experiences and affirms being connected in oneness with both nurse and nursed as caring is lived in the moment.

Gayle entered into Tracy's world that night open to hearing a special call. Gayle's openness was partly a reflection of her use of the empirical pathway of knowing, the data given in report, the comparison of empirical observations against biological, psychological, developmental, and social norms. Before discussing our understanding of Gayle's response from the theoretical perspective presented, it might be helpful to compare how the call for nursing may have been interpreted if approached, for example, from a psychological framework. If the nurse responded from a psychological framework, the problem identified would perhaps be conceptualized as *denial* on the part of Tracy's mother. It could be assumed that Tracy's mother was avoiding the reality of the impending death of her daughter. Here, the nursing goal would be to assist the mother in dealing with her denial by facilitating grieving. Denial is only one psychological concept that could be applied in this situation; avoidance, anxiety, and loss are others. When nursing care is *based* on a psychological framework, however, the central theme of care is likely to be de-emphasized in favor of a problem-oriented approach. The perspective offered by a normative discipline requires a reliance on empirical knowing. Using only the empirical pathway of knowing, the richness of nursing is lost.

Gayle's personal knowing, her intuition, however, was the pathway that illuminated the appreciation of this situation and prompted her acknowledgement of a call. She heard Tracy's call for the intimacy, comfort, and protection of her mother's presence as she (Tracy) summoned courage and hope for her journey. Gayle intuitively knew that the specific caring being called forth was the caring of a mother. Gayle's caring response also took the form of the courageous acknowledgement of a call for nursing that would be difficult to substantiate empirically. Beyond telephoning Tracy's mother, Gayle continued her nursing effort to answer Tracy's call for the presence of a mother as she supported Mrs. P. living her interconnectedness, in being with Tracy. Gayle heard Mrs. P.'s calls for knowing, knowing what to do and knowing that it would be right to do it, for the courage to be with her daughter in this new difficult passage. Her response of showing the way reflects hope and humility. The caring between the nurse and the ones nursed enhanced the personhood of all three, as each grew in caring ways. It is possible that the caring between the original participants in the nursing situation and those of us who are participating through engagement with the text continues to enhance personhood.

REFERENCES

Boykin, A., & Schoenhofer, S. (1991). Story as link between nursing practice, ontology, epistemology. *Image, 23,* 245–248.

Boykin, A., & Schoenhofer, S. (1990). Caring in nursing: Analysis of extant theory. *Nursing Science Quarterly, 4,* 149–155.

Maxwell, G. (1990). Connections. *Nightingale Songs, 1*(1). P.O. Box 057563, West Palm Beach, FL 33405).

Paterson, J., & Zderad, L. (1988). *Humanistic nursing.* New York: National League for Nursing Press.

Roach, S. (1984). *Caring: The human mode of being, implications for nursing.* Toronto: Faculty of Nursing, University of Toronto. (Perspectives in Caring Monograph 1).

Schoenhofer, S. (1989). Love, beauty and truth: Fundamental nursing values. *Journal of Nursing Education, 28*(8), 382–384.

Watson, J. (1987). Nursing on the caring edge; Metaphorical vignettes. *Advances in Nursing Science, 10,* 10–18.

4

IMPLICATIONS FOR PRACTICE AND NURSING SERVICE ADMINISTRATION

*F*oundations for practice of the Nursing as Caring theory rest on the nurse coming to know self as caring person in ever deepening and broadening dimensions. While all nurses may have (or at least, may have had) a sense of self as caring person, practicing within this theoretical framework requires a deliberate commitment to developing this knowledge. In many settings where nurses find themselves practicing, there is little in the environment to support a commitment to ongoing development of a sense of self as caring person. In fact, many practice environments seem to support knowing self only as instrument, self as technology. When one perceives of one's "nursing self" as a depersonalized, disembodied tool, nursing tends to lose its flavor and the devoted commitment to nursing burns out. So how to sustain and actualize this fundamental commitment must be a point of serious study for the nurse who desires to practice nursing as caring.

Mayeroff's (1971) caring ingredients are useful tools to assist the nurse in developing an ever-present awareness of self as caring person. Taking note of personal patterns of expressing hope, honesty, courage, and the other ingredients is a good starting place. Understanding the meaning of living caring in one's own life is an important base for practicing nursing as caring. In reflecting on a particular lived experience of caring, the nurse can seek to understand the ways in which caring contributed freedom within the situation—freedom to be, freedom to choose, and freedom to unfold.

Because nursing *is* a way of living caring in the world, the nurse can turn his or her attention to personal patterns of nursing as expressions of caring. As self understanding as caring person accrues, the nurse sometimes realizes that such self-awareness was there all along—it was only waiting to be discovered. Because many nurses were trained to overlook their caring ways instead of attending to them, nurses may now need something similar to, or indeed "sensitivity train-ing" itself, to rediscover and reown the possibilities of self as caring person, possibilities specific to nursing as a profession and a discipline. This redirection of focus away from caring may have been related to several historical social movements. First, of course, is the move toward science, which for nursing meant that for a period of several decades nursing educators seemed to reject, either partially or totally, the art of nursing in order to discover a scientific base for practice. Another re-lated process, the technology movement, led nurses to under-stand care as a series of sequential actions designed to accomplish a specifiable end. In this context, nursing care became synonymous with managing available technologies. Third, there existed in the history of nursing education an era(s) in which nurses were taught to treat symptoms patients expressed, rather than to care for the person. Fourth, main-taining a professional distance was a hallmark of professional-ism. Now, and rightly so, the tide has turned. A reawakening of knowing self as caring person becomes paramount so that the profession of nursing returns caring to the immediacy of the nursing situation.

With personal awareness and reflection, developed knowledge of caring also arrives through empirical, ethical, and aesthetic modes of knowing. There is a growing body of literature in nursing that both attests to that fact and to the process of how nurses communicate caring in practice (e.g., Riemen, 1986a; 1986b; Knowlden, 1986; Swanson-Kauffman, 1986a, 1986b; Swanson, 1990; Kahn and Steeves, 1988). Given the various perspectives offered by the authors just mentioned, the individual nurse can enhance his or her ethical self-devel-opment as caring person by cultivating the practice of weigh-ing the various meanings of caring now extant in actual practice situations and then by making choices to express car-ing creatively. In pursuit of this end, aesthetic knowing often subsumes and transcends other forms of knowing and thus may offer the richest mode of knowing caring. Appreciating structure, form, harmony, and complementarity across a range of situated caring expressions enhances knowing self and other as caring persons.

Knowing self as caring enhances knowing of the other as caring. Knowing other as caring contributes to our discovery of caring self. Without knowing the other as caring person, there can be no true nursing. Living a commitment to nursing as caring can be a tremendous challenge when nurses are asked to care for someone who makes it difficult to care. In effect, it is impossible to avoid the issue of "liking" or "disliking" the patient. Is it possible to truly care for someone if the nurse doesn't like him or her? In this light, another question arises: How can I enter the world of another who repulses me? Am I expected to pretend that this person (the patient) has not treated others inhumanely (if that is the case)? Must I ignore the reality of the other's hatefulness toward me (if such exists)? These are questions that come from the human heart. They express legitimate human issues that present themselves regularly in nursing situations.

The commitment of the nurse practicing nursing as caring is to nurture persons living caring and growing in caring. Again, this implies that the nurse come to know the other as caring person *in the moment.* "Difficult to care" situations are those that demonstrate the extent of knowledge and commitment needed to nurse effectively. An everyday understanding of the meaning of caring is obviously inadequate when the nurse is presented with someone for whom it is difficult to care. In these extreme (though not unusual) situations, a task-oriented, nondiscipline-based concept of nursing may be adequate to assure the completion of certain treatment and surveillance techniques. Still, in our eyes that is an insufficient response—it certainly is not the nursing we advocate. The theory, Nursing as Caring, calls upon the nurse to reach deep within a well-developed knowledge base that has been structured using all available patterns of knowing, grounded in the obligations inherent in the commitment to know persons as caring. These patterns of knowing may include intuition, scientifically quantifiable data emerging from research, related knowledge from a variety of disciplines, ethical beliefs, as well as many other types of knowing. All knowledge held by the nurse which may be relevant to understanding the situation at hand is drawn forward and integrated into practice in particular nursing situations. Although the degree of challenge presented from situation to situation varies, the commitment to know self and other as caring persons is steadfast.

Caring expressed in nursing is personal, not abstract. The caring that is nursing cannot be expressed as an impersonal generalized stance of good will, but must be expressed knowledgeably. That is, the caring that is nursing must be a lived experience of caring, communicated intentionally, and in authentic presence through a person-with-person interconnectedness, a sense of oneness with self and other. The nurse is not expected to be super-human, superficial, or naive. Rather, a genuine openness to caring and a formed intention of knowing the other as caring person are required. In this sense, and referring back to patients with whom an expression of empathy is problematic, liking may be understood as a less personally committed form of caring or loving. In other words, liking is superficial and may not require the devotion needed to know other as caring. When the nurse truly connects with the other, liking the other becomes a moot issue.

Stories nurses tell about their nursing bring to light the sustenance they find in the nursing situation. Lived experiences of practice, recounted to crystallize the essential meaning of nursing, contain the tangible seeds of awareness of self as caring person. However, the nurse may not be fully aware of self as caring person until the nursing story is *articulated* and *shared*. When the practicing nurse can begin to describe practice as the personal expression of caring with and for another, possibilities for living nursing as caring emerge.

Here is one nurse's response to the invitation to tell a story that conveys the beauty of nursing. The authentic presence of the nurse in the following nursing situation focuses on honesty as an expression of self as caring person.

HONESTY

As Jason came through the door to RAC, a young black man lying lifelessly on a stretcher of pale green linen, the surgeon came towards me telling me *not* to tell Jason that his biopsy was positive.

I felt inner terror. A man, less than 18 years old, was going to come close to the "truth" of living today. Yet the terror inside me was really fueled by the becoming moral issue I was *going to face soon.*

Jason was surely going to ask of the results upon waking from anesthesia. "They always do." Going to sleep unknowing demands waking-to-know. "Honesty."

Honesty as a lived precept of caring requires that I, nurse, must always and ever regard the person nursed from a position of love. I must enter all nursing activity with the sole purpose of using truth, only and ever, to promote the spiritual growth of the person nursed. In this climate of openness to myself and to the other, we can begin to experience freedom from fear.

Jason inevitably opened his eyes only seconds or minutes later—I was so concerned with the surgeon's directive I lost perception of time. My choice? The surgeon's choice? Jason's choice?

All too soon, before I could decide "how" to act, Jason had arrived at our moment of honesty versus dishonesty.

There were tears in Jason's eyes and as quickly as the endotracheal tube was removed, words came from Jason's essence. "Why me, God?"

I was pre-empted. (That's what happens when *I* write the script of nursing.)

Instead of dancing around "telling" Jason, I was now only able to "be-with" Jason. To suffer with Jason, to come to compassionate knowing of Jason's subjective reality.

"I heard him," Jason choked and sobbed.

I just sat next to his stretcher and held his left hand with my right hand. I softly stroked his shoulder. This intimate hand-in-hand gesture only expressed a small part of the instant connectedness that we were co-experiencing, each alone, each with the other, *all at once.*

I sat there for more than thirty minutes telling Jason repeatedly to rest, trust God to help him, have strength, courage, and hope.

Having come together, Jason and I, through the darkness of anesthetized sleep to the harsh reality of "wakefulness," we must both move on with our lives.

I asked the surgeon of Jason several times, but he couldn't remember Jason.

I will never forget Jason. Jason brought me closer to understanding honesty as caring (Little, 1992).

An explicit realization of nursing as a personal expression of caring can fuel a commitment to growing in caring throughout life. A vivid, articulated sense of self connects with an equally strong and explicit sense of nursing, and a personal commitment to caring in and through nursing is created. Research makes the unequivocal point that those who seek our nursing service identify caring as the sine qua non of nursing (Samaral, 1988; Winland-Brown & Schoenhofer, 1992). Entering these covenantal relationships obligates us to mutually live and grow in caring. What has also become apparent through our practice is that it is increasingly difficult for nurses to conceptualize their service as caring. Many nurses have lost faith in themselves as persons contributing caring in health service delivery situations. Thus, the raison d'etre for the professional service career of nursing is lost, and nurses become disheartened.

It is our experience, as illustrated in the previous story, *Honesty,* that nurses can recapture the spirit of nursing, can rekindle hope for themselves as persons caring through and in nursing. The reader is invited to pause a moment and experience a sense of self as person expressing caring in nursing.

> You are invited to enter a quiet, contemplative inner space. Allow the attentions and distractions of the moment to recede as you create quietude. Now, bring to life the most beautiful nursing you have ever done. Recall that precious instance that stands out for you as *truly nursing.* Savor the fullness of that experience. Explore the meaning of this wonderful experience of nursing.
>
> If possible, pause now and tell the story of your finest nursing moment—aloud to another nurse, or in writing to the nurse you are today. Share your story and invite other nurses to share theirs with you.
>
> Now that the moment has been reborn and communicated, it is available as a powerful resource for you. The essence of nursing which connects you to all others in nursing is also to be found here. In that story resides the central meaning of nursing, available now for your inspiration and for your study.

For many nurses, the practice of nursing as caring will require changes in the conceptualization of nursing and nursing practice structures. Certain ideologies and cognitive frameworks that have gained prominence in nursing in the recent past are not fully congruent with the values expressed in the Nursing as Caring theory.

For example, the problem-solving process introduced into nursing by Orlando (1961), known as the Nursing Process, comes from a worldview that is incompatible with that which undergirds nursing as caring. In the 1960s, nurses came to value Orlando's Nursing Process for its role in helping them organize and put to use a growing body of scientific nursing knowledge. Having borrowed the "problematizing" approach to service delivery that was so successful in medical contexts, the Nursing Process also fit with an emerging documentation system known as Problem Oriented Medical Records, which again was adapted from medicine for nursing use. During the late 1970s and through the 1980s, this impetus was further developed in the Nursing Diagnosis movement.

What difficulties exist with the problem-solving process in nursing? More than anything else, this process directs nurses to locate something in the internal or external environment or character of the client that is in need of correction. Gadow (1984) refers to this view as a paradigm of philanthropy. In this demeaning paradigm, "touch is a gift from one who is whole to one who is not" (p. 68). Within the context of Orlando's Nursing Process, such problem-solving requires that the nurse first find something that needs correction to legitimately offer appropriate care. This focus on correction—and cure—both distracts nurses from their primary mission of caring and therefore practice results in objectification, labeling, ritualism, and non-involvement. The context for nursing is lost.

Further, the Orlando's Process has resulted in nursing's knowledge base being ever more deeply grounded in disciplines other than nursing. An examination of a list of nursing diagnoses reveals that specific knowledge from disciplines such as medicine, psychology, anthropology, sociology, and epidemiology is what is required to solve the problems to which the diagnoses refer. Rather than leading nurses toward the development of the knowledge of nursing, Orlando's Nursing Process has intensified the concept of nursing as a context-free integrator of other disciplines.

The following story of a nursing situation demonstrates the freedom and creativity that is possible when the nurse takes a focused, unfolding view of the lived world of nursing. What occasioned this nursing relationship was conceptualized in the larger system as providing care for the caregiver, providing support in a family context. Here, home nursing is seen as once again on the ascendancy as nurses discover what is increasingly missing in institutional bureaucratic settings— the opportunity to nurse.

CONNECTEDNESS

I was with J. tonight, and for the first time *I* enjoyed "authentic presence" with her. I am not so sure it was because I was less fatigued and more receptive to "what is" in her home, but because J. was clearly "different" tonight. She greeted me with her usual rush of activity and then startled me by asking me to "be with me, please," when she gave her son an injection and changed the injection site on his central venous catheter line. I had met her son before, but had never been invited to his room or the upstairs quarters. We spent a long time in A's room with J. and A. talking, sharing thoughts and feelings about (sister) K., frustrations of J. trying to do it all and still find a little peaceful time for herself, angry outbursts and feelings of shame and sadness, and J's desire to go to Mass on Sunday without feelings of extreme anger and despair because K. cries when J. leaves the house, and ending with J's stated determination to do the impossible task of being all things to all people at all times. The dialogue was really between mother and son, with questions directed toward me but immediately answered by J. and A. The conversation was sparkling with humor and piercing with honesty, and created in my mind's eye a rich, colorful mosaic of years of love, beauty, and truth. Tonight I wish I were an artist so I could capture this vision on canvas.

J. asked me to stay with A. while she did a small chore in the kitchen, and I settled in a side chair for whatever might present itself. The I.V. pole in the corner of the room caught my attention and A. offered the name of the drug and its purpose. I honestly did not know that particular drug, and had nothing to offer, so I just nodded my head. A. looked at me, cleared his throat, and proceeded to tell me about a problem he is encountering. I interrupted him and told him that I know nothing about him other than his name and he is J's son, and that J. has not shared anything about him privately with me. He smiled, and then with his head bowed and eyes peering at me, told me that he has AIDS, worries about the stigma, and dreads the stance most health professionals assume when he encounters them as they interpret the name of his disease process. I sat very still and nodded my head. I wanted to acknowledge his pain and show acceptance of him and what appeared to be his need to connect with me. Together we reflected on the wonderfulness of the human spirit, the concept of personhood, and holistic beings with thoughts, feelings, wants, and needs. When A. was ready we ventured down the stairs and found J. sitting quietly in a rocking chair. It seemed she had finished her "task," and I wondered how long she had been sitting alone. I sensed that she had invited me into her private pain, and courageously shared another part of her life with me. I also knew intuitively that she did not want to talk about it.

J. had prepared the piano, and all of them asked me to play for them and expressed disappointment that I did not play the piano during my visit last week. So I played gentle, reflective songs interspersed with light melodic phrases. Requests were offered by each member of the family, and within minutes J. was sitting next to me on the piano bench, singing loudly and punctuating words with feelings and strength and lending incredible meaning to lyrics. "Old Man River," deep, low, rumbling of the piano and purposefully driving tempo was responded to in kind with J. stamping her foot with each beat and pounding her knee with each word as she emphatically sang "He just keeps rolling along, he keeps on rolling along." It seemed to be cathartic for her as expressions seemed to come from the center of her being. We applauded ourselves when we finished and J. let me hug her. A. caught my eye and mouthed "thank you for helping my mother to smile." J. was quiet then, and I felt her exhaustion. We agreed that it was time to close the piano for another week, and I left. J. followed me to my car, and left me with "God bless you."

This was an exhausting visit to J's home, yet it was even more energizing because of the multiple caring moments I experienced with J. and her family. I have come to believe that caring moments are unique to each nursing situation and evolve naturally from the mutuality of authentic presence as the fullness of the nurse's personhood blends with the fullness of the other's personhood. Together they transcend the moment. The caring moment is connectedness between nurse and other and both experience moments of joy. (Kronk, 1992)

To characterize this nursing situation with a nursing diagnosis and to portray it as a linear process driven by the diagnosis or problem to be addressed with a pre-envisioned outcome would be to rob the situation of all the beauty of nursing. Because a story of a nursing situation is narrative, there is a temporal structure. However, this structure supports rather than destroys the "lived experience" character of the situation. The story of the nursing situation conveys the "all-at-once" as well as the unfolding. This approach permits us to conceptualize as well as contextualize the knowledge of nursing the story tells. Through story, the meaning for this nurse of knowing herself as caring person, as entering into the world of other(s) with authentic presence, is understood. The nurse knows other as caring person, and in that knowing attends to specific calls for caring with unique expressions of caring responses created in the moment.

The Nursing as Caring theory, grounded in the assumption that all persons are caring, has as its focus a general call to nurture persons as they live caring uniquely and grow as caring persons. The challenge then for nursing is not to discover what is missing, weakened, or needed in another, but to come to know the other as caring person and to nurture that person in situation-specific, creative ways. We no longer understand nursing as a "process," in the sense of a complex sequence of predictable acts resulting in some predetermined desirable end product. Nursing is, we believe, *processual,* in the sense that it is always unfolding and that it is guided by intention.

Nursing is a professional service offered in social contexts, most often in bureaucratically organized health services. Discussions of health services, overheard in boardrooms and legislative chambers, are languaged in impersonal, aggregate, disembodying, and perhaps more importantly, economic terms. In contrast to the accepted ritualization of such language, nursing has a very important role to play—to bring the *human,* the *personal* dimension to health policy planning, and health care delivery systems. Clearly, it is nursing knowledge itself, of human person, of person as caring, that has been missing. While other groups rightly bring in knowledge of efficient operation and financing, nursing's contribution to the dialogue on effective care has the potential to remind all players of the real bottom line, the person being cared for. We must remember that in most industrialized countries health service is viewed as a commodity delivery system, an economic exchange of goods and services. While this is not the only context for nursing, it is the most prevalent context. If nurses choose to participate in existing delivery systems, and most do, then ways must be created that preserve the service of nursing while responding to the appropriate requirements of the system. Ultimately, this would require of nurses that they become skilled in articulating their service as nursing, and connecting that service to the recording and billing systems in use. Although this same goal animated the nursing diagnosis movement of the 1970s, within the terms of that movement, the result was less than fortunate: nursing's effort to emulate the fee-for-service billing practices of medicine failed, and nursing contributions were neither communicated nor reimbursed.

When nurses tell the stories of their nursing situations, however, the service of nursing becomes recognizable. The unique contribution that nurses make, expressed in the focus of nursing, emerges across settings. The difference between a nursing story and a typical nursing case report is striking; the first conveys the nursing care given, the second reports the medical-assisting activities performed by the nurse. We have discovered in our work with nurses that while nursing care is usually given, it is frequently neither acknowledged nor communicated.

The nurse practicing within the caring context described here will most often be interfacing with the health care system in two ways: first, to communicate nursing in ways that can be understood; and second, to articulate nursing service as a unique contribution within the system in such a way that the system itself grows to support nursing.

The concept of *profession* is involved in the practice of nursing as caring. With the advent of the information and action technologies of the twenty-first century, the present concept of professions as repositories of esoteric knowledge employed by social elites is rapidly becoming outdated. As many nurses will attest, the patient often teaches the nurse about new medical technologies and about the management of them. In this regard, what will it mean, in the next century, to profess nursing? A renewed commitment to professing caring means that nurses would seek connectedness in all collegial relationships as nurses are open to discovering the unfolding meaning of human caring, with persons valued as important in themselves. Therefore, nurses forfeit assuming authoritative stances toward each other, the persons nursed, and other participants in the health care enterprise. More than ever, it will mean that nurses will, in relation with others, live out the value of caring in everyday life. Thus, the organized nursing profession would assume responsibility for developing and sharing knowledge of nurturing persons living caring and growing in caring.

The following story of a nursing situation, told in the form of a poem, exemplifies the reconceptualization called for in the practice of Nursing as Caring. In this situation, the nurse carried out a medically prescribed treatment, not as a form of medicine but as a form of nursing. The nurse communicates a knowing of the other as caring person, living courage and hope in the face of pain and fear. This example illustrates the meaning of knowing as a caring ingredient (Mayeroff, 1971), in the connectedness of the nurse with the patient. The nurse's knowing both forms the intention to nurse and is formed by the intention to know other as caring person and nurture caring. A more typical recounting of this situation would focus on the specific procedure of the treatment being applied, in terms of the condition of the wound. In this poem, the nurse renders the meaning of nursing.

HEALING—HIV+

Your wounds weeped
Purulent with the discharge of our
Pain and fear.
They tried to hide, only to reappear.
The treatment gentle, slow
A warm, loving balm to your soul.
Your stomach was fed the comfort
Food of your youth
And your lips drank in deeply all
You knew and understood.
The memories sweetened each moment
You stood, face to face with terror of
What might be mistook.
All inside shifted as slowly it came,
A gradual awakening; embracing of pain
As you conquered your demons
A lightness appeared
To stay forever and
Abolish all fears. (Wheeler, 1990)

NURSING SERVICE ADMINISTRATION

Many of the nursing situations described in this book have taken place in hospital settings, where the nursing service is a shared responsibility of many nurses in a range of functional roles. Nurses in such settings generally nurse many persons intensively and simultaneously and share direct nursing responsibility with one or two other nurses. How can nurses in institutional practice settings be supported so that calls for nursing can be heard and nursing responses made? What is the role of the nurse administrator in supporting the practice of nurses?

It is important to understand clearly the difference between the practice of administration which happens to be delivered by nurses and the practice of nursing administration. Tead (1951) defines administration as "the comprehensive effort to direct, guide, and integrate associated human strivings which are focused toward some specific ends or aims" (p. 3). For example, goals of administration could be business, governmental, education, or nursing. In this definition, it is evident that the focus must be made clear. It is not adequate to have an understanding of administration as a role which is focused in functions such as interpersonal, informational, and decisional. Such a perspective ignores the value of persons and the ministering responsibilities inherent in the role. The administrator must connect his or her work to the direct work of nursing.

Nursing administration by name suggests a groundedness in the discipline. The role of the nursing administrator could indeed be questioned if the focus of the administrative practice is not nursing. There is the assumption that the administration of nursing is practiced from a particular conception of nursing in which the focus or goal of nursing is clear. What the nursing administrator says and does as nurse must reflect the uniqueness of the discipline so that nursing's unique contributions are assured. Nursing administrators must also be able to articulate the unique contributions of nursing to other members of the interdisciplinary health care team.

The relationship of the nurse administrator's role to direct care is implicit in this perspective. The nursing administrator describes him or herself as directly involved in the care of persons. All activities of the nursing administrator are ultimately directed to the person(s) being nursed. It is essential that this direct connection to the goal of nursing be made and that persons assuming nursing administration positions be able to articulate their unique role contributions to nursing care. Without this clarity of focus, one may be engaged in the practice of administration but not nursing administration.

From the viewpoint of nursing as caring, the nurse administrator makes decisions through a lens in which the focus of nursing is nurturing persons as they live caring and grow in caring. All activities in the practice of nursing administration are grounded in a concern for creating, maintaining, and supporting an environment in which calls for nursing are heard and nurturing responses are given. From this point of view, the expectation arises that nursing administrators participate in shaping a culture that evolves from the values articulated within nursing as caring.

Although often perceived to be "removed" from the direct care of the nursed, the nursing administrator is intimately involved in multiple nursing situations simultaneously, hearing calls for nursing and participating in responses to these calls. As calls for nursing are known, one of the unique responses of the nursing administrator is to directly or indirectly enter the world of the nursed, understand special calls when they occur, and assist in securing the resources needed by the nurse to nurture persons as they live and grow in caring. All nursing activities should be approached with this goal in mind. Here, the nurse administrator reflects on the obligations inherent in the role in relation to the nursed. The presiding moral basis for determining right action is the belief that all persons are caring. Frequently, the nurse administrator may enter the world of the nursed through the stories of colleagues who are assuming other roles such as nurse manager. Policy formulation and implementation allow for the consideration of unique situations. The nursing administrator assists others within the organization to understand the focus of nursing and to secure the resources necessary to achieve the goals of nursing. When the focus of nursing can be clearly articulated, nursing's contribution to the whole will be understood. If the focus of practice is clouded, however, this becomes an insurmountable task. Recognition of nursing's value is contingent upon the ability of nurses to articulate their contribution. Traditionally, systems define contribution through patient outcomes and other total quality measures. Future articulation of nursing and its contributions would emanate from the values and assumptions offered in the Nursing as Caring theory.

Sharing nursing situations with others is one way to promote the knowing of nursing. It also is a way for other members of the organization to see how their roles contribute to the well-being of the nursed. The following is a nursing situation, re-presented as the poem "Last Rights," that cries out for nursing administration, that is, nursing support for nursing.

LAST RIGHTS

Tight faced, they found and cornered her at work
As quick as hammers pounding down a wall
of words came hard and nailed that little quirk
of honesty so fast she held the rail.

"Who were you to say he was a dying
man, though he lay white, his lifethread thin.
How were you to know the speed his flying
heart would race away from bone and skin.

He was hopeless, yes, beneath that tent
of filmy gauze, but who were you to say
his fate was hinged in prayer—our magic spent.
Who knows, he might have lived another day.

He held my hands and asked the truth," she said.
Then turned away to smooth the empty bed.

Yelland-Marino (1993)

The nurse administrator can nurture the living in caring and growing in caring of the person in this story by creating ways to support the nurse at the bedside in order that the call for hope of being known and supported as caring person, not object, can occur. What are some of the strategies that the nurse administrator could engage in which would reflect the nursing focus?

Because budget determination is such a prominent matter for nurse administrators, we will begin there. Budget decisions should be directed from the perspective of what I ought to do as nurse administrator that would have the greatest effect on nurturing persons being cared for in their living and growing in caring. One aspect of budget essential to this story is time—time for the nurse to focus on knowing self and other colleagues. As Paterson & Zderad (1988) state, for nursing practice to be humanistic, awareness of self and others is essential. The budget should include time allocations for staff to participate in dialogues focused on knowing self as caring person in order that calls, such as the one in the previous story, can be heard. The notion of dialogue is central to transforming ways of being with others in organizations. Bohm (1992) refers to dialogue as creating "a flow of meaning in the whole group, out of which will emerge some new understanding, something creative" (p. 16). Persons engaged in dialogue are focused on trying to understand situations as perceived through another's eyes in order that new possibilities may be recognized. Through the allocation of time, nursing staff come to better know self and other. Shared meanings emerge which become the "glue or cement that holds people and societies together" (p. 16). These opportunities for knowing self assist the nurse to achieve, as Tournier (1957) would put it, a reciprocity of consciousness with other.

Through the opportunity to better know self as caring person, the nurse will learn to intentionally and authentically enter nursing situations focused on knowing and supporting the nursed as they live caring and grow in caring. Time for reflection and collegial dialogue is necessary to maintain this nursing lens in a period of increasing responsibility. Such time allocation communicates the commitment of the nurse administrator to enhance the growth of the nurse in the discipline of nursing.

To propose that the budgeting of time is one of the most essential tasks of a nursing administrator may seem outrageously naive in a time when organizations seem to be interested only in bottom-line figures. Ironically, however, the time allocation strategy offered here supports the goal of cost containment. Studies have shown that caring behaviors of nurses (Duffy, 1991) and nursing staff attitudes (Cassarea et al., 1986) are directly related to patient satisfaction. Benner and Wrubel (1989) also found that caring is integral to expert practice. As a result, and from the standpoint of quality of care as revenue producing, this strategy of allowing time for dialogue and reflection has merit.

From the viewpoint of the Nursing as Caring theory, the nurse administrator's beliefs about person would require that new ways of being with the nursed are created and supported. The nursing administrator models a way of being with others that portrays respect for person as caring. Through modeling, others grow in their competency to know and express caring. Of course creating and sustaining environments that nurture and value the practice and study of nursing remains the challenge facing nurses caught in the maze of various organizational structures. Systems tend to perpetuate existing ways of being even though their members may repeatedly question the legitimacy of actions flowing from these structures. It is our belief that nursing can create a culture that values caring within systems and organizations. Systems and organizations can be reshaped and transformed through living out the assumptions and values inherent within nursing as caring.

Assumptions on which Nursing as Caring is built serve as stabilizers for the organization. These assumptions directly influence the climate of the organization and serve as the organizational pillars. The climate of organizations is determined by beliefs and values of persons within it. An organization grounded in the assumptions of person as described in Chapter 1 would not support arbitrary and capricious decision making in which the input of all persons has not been discerned. Mission statements, goals, objectives, standards of practice, policies and procedures emerge from assumptions, beliefs, and values that emphasize one's humanness. If one accepts the assumption that persons are caring by virtue of their humanness, then it follows that cultures are comprised of caring persons. Respect for person as person is engendered within this context. There is a desire to know and support the living of caring; to support each other in being who we are as caring persons in the moment. Therefore, assumptions of Nursing as Caring ground not only the theory but may likewise influence the ontology of the organization itself.

Generally, organizational structures reflect bureaucratic values. Structures imply ways of being with and relating to people. The process of relating is typically illustrated in a hierarchical fashion. The concept of hierarchy carries with it the notion that there is a "top" and a "bottom." Competition, levels, and positions of power are implicit. In climbing the rungs of a bureaucratic ladder, it is difficult for the employee to be authentic and valued as a unique person with special ideas because the risks of such valuing are often too great for the bureaucracy to bear. Competition too remains the driving force of most organizations.

Within an organization, however, we can imagine each person's hands as clinging to the rungs of the bureaucratic ladder. Taken further, this image would clearly portray persons who are not and can not be open to receive and know other. Because of the vertical axis of the bureaucratic hierarchy, persons, more often than not, are viewed as objects. The ladder positions people so that they are either looking up or down but rarely eye-to-eye. Obviously, the hierarchical model does not support the idea of each person as important in and to him or herself.

By contrast, and from the assumptions posited in Nursing as Caring, the model for being in relationships resembles a dance of caring persons (Boykin, 1990). The same persons are present in this circle that were in the hierarchical structure described above. The difference between the two models is the philosophical way of being with other. Because the nature of relating in the circle is grounded in a respect for and valuing of each person, the way of being is diametrically opposed to traditional patterns of relating in organizations. Leaving the security provided by known hierarchical structures, however, requires courage, trust, and humility. Building on the assumptions of this theory, one can infer that the basic dance of all persons in relationships is to know self and other as caring person. Relationships are transformed through knowing and valuing other as caring person. Each person is encouraged and supported in a culture that values person-as-person, person as caring.

The image of a dancing circle is also used to describe being for and being with the nursed. In the circle, all persons are committed to knowing self and other as living and growing in caring. Each dancer makes a distinct contribution because of

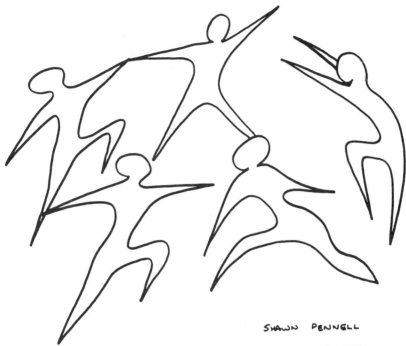

SHAWN PENNELL

THE DANCE OF CARING PERSONS

the role assumed. The dancers in the circle do not necessarily connect by holding hands although they may. Each dancer moves within this dance as called forth by the nature of the nursing situation. The nursed calls for services of particular dancers at various points in time. Each person is in this circle because of their unique contribution to the person being cared for . . . nurses, administrators, human resources, etc. These roles would not exist if it were not for the nursed. There is always room for another person to join the dance. Rather than the vertical view described earlier, this model fosters knowing other. Eye-to-eye contact assists one to know and appreciate each other as caring persons. Each person is viewed as special and caring. No one person's role is more or less important than the other's. Each role is essential in contributing to the process of living grounded in caring. As each person authentically expresses their commitment in being there for and with the nursed, caring relationships are lived. When the focus in any health care institution fails to be the person cared-for, purpose, roles, and responsibilities become depersonalized and bureaucratic rather than person-centered and caring.

Personal knowing—knowing of self and other—is integral to the connectedness of persons in this dance. The nursing administrator interfaces with persons of many disciplines as well as with the nursed. With each interaction, the nurse administrator is honest and authentic in encouraging others to know and live out who they are. Each encounter with another is an opportunity for knowing other as caring person. From an organizational standpoint the nursing administrator assists in creating a community that appreciates, nurtures, and supports each person as they live and grow in caring moment to moment. The nursing administrator assists nurses to hear and understand the unique calls for nursing and supports and sustains their nurturing responses.

REFERENCES

Benner, P., & Wrubel, J. (1989). *The primacy of caring: Stress and coping in health and illness.* CA: Addison-Wesley.

Bohm, D. (1992). On dialogue. *Noetic Sciences Review,* pp. 16–18.

Boykin, A. (1990). Creating a caring environment: Moral obligations in role of dean. In M. Leininger & J. Watson (Eds.), *The caring imperative in education.* New York: National League for Nursing, pp. 247–254.

Cassarrea, K., Mills, J., & Plant, M. (1986). Improving service through patient surveys in a multihospital organization. *Hospital and Health Services Administration, 31*(2), 41–52.

Duffy, J. (1992). The impact of nurse caring on patient outcomes. In Gaut, D. (Ed.). *The presence of caring in nursing.* New York: National League for Nursing, pp. 113–136.

Gadow, S. (1984). Touch and technology: Two paradigms of patient care. *Journal of Religion and Health, 23,* 63–69.

Kahn, D., & Steeves, R. (1988). Caring and practice: Construction of the nurse's world. *Scholarly Inquiry for Nursing Practice, 2*(3), 201–215.

Knowlden, V. (1986). The meaning of caring in the nursing role. *Dissertation Abstracts International, 46*(9), 2574-A.

Kronk, P. (1992). *Connectedness: A concept for nursing.* Unpublished manuscript.

Little, D. (1992). *Nurse as moral agent.* Paper presented at University of South Florida Year of Discovery Seminar, Sept. 1992.

Mayeroff, M. (1971). *On caring.* New York: Harper & Row.

Orlando, I. (1961). *The dynamic nurse-patient relationship.* New York: G. P. Putnam's Sons.

Paterson, J., & Zderad, L. (1988). *Humanistic nursing.* New York: National League for Nursing.

Riemen, D. (1986a). Noncaring and caring in the clinical setting: Patients' descriptions. *Topics in Clinical Nursing, 8,* 30–36.

Riemen, D. (1986b). The essential structure of a caring interaction: doing phenomenology. In P. Munhall & C. Oiler (Eds.). *Nursing research: A qualitative perspective.* Norwalk, CT: Appleton-Century-Crofts.

Roach, S. (1987). *The human act of caring.* Ottawa: Canadian Hospital Association.

Samarel, N. (1988). Caring for life and death: Nursing in a hospital-based hospice. *Dissertation abstracts international, 48*(9), 2607-B.

Swanson-Kauffman, K. (1986a). Caring in the instance of un-expected early pregnancy loss. *Topics in Clinical Nursing, 8,* 37–46.

Swanson-Kauffman, K. (1986b). A combined qualitative methodology for nursing research. *Advances in Nursing Science, 8,* 58–69.

Swanson, K. (1990). Providing care in the NICU: Sometimes an act of love. *Advances in Nursing Science, 13*(1), 60–73.

Tead, O. (1951). *The art of administration.* New York: McGraw-Hill.

Tournier, P. (1957). *The meaning of persons.* New York: Harper & Row.

Wheeler, L. (1990). Healing-HIV+. *Nightingale Songs,* P. O. Box 057563, West Palm Beach, FL 33405-7563, *1*(2).

Winland-Brown, J., & Schoenhofer, S. (1992). Unpublished research data.

Yelland-Marino, T. (1993). Last rights. *Nightingale Songs,* P. O. Box 057563, West Palm Beach, FL 33405-7563, *3*(1).

5

IMPLICATIONS FOR NURSING EDUCATION

*I*n this chapter, we address the implications of our theory for nursing education, including designing, implementing, and administering a program of study. The assumptions that ground Nursing as Caring also ground the practice of nursing education and nursing education administration. The structure and practices of the education program are expressions of the discipline and, therefore, should be explicit reflections of the values and assumptions inherent in the statement of focus of the discipline. From the perspective of Nursing as Caring, all structures and activities should reflect the fundamental assumption that persons are caring by virtue of their humanness. Other assumptions and values reflected in the education program include: knowing the person as whole and complete in the moment and living caring uniquely; understanding that personhood is a process of living grounded in caring and is enhanced through participation in nurturing relationships with caring others; and, finally, affirming nursing as a discipline and profession.

The curriculum, the foundation of the education program, asserts the focus and domain of nursing as nurturing persons living caring and growing in caring. All activities of the program of study are directed toward developing, organizing, and communicating nursing knowledge, that is, knowledge of nurturing persons living caring and growing in caring.

The model for organizational design of nursing education is analogous to the dancing circle described earlier. Members of the circle include administrators, faculty, colleagues, students, staff, community, and the nursed. What this circle represents is the commitment of each dancer to understanding and supporting the study of the discipline of nursing. The role of administrator in the circle is more clearly understood when the origin of the word is reflected upon. The term *administrator* derives from the Latin *ad ministrare,* to serve (Guralnik,

1976). This definition connotes the idea of rendering service. Administrators within the circle are by nature of role obligated to ministering, to securing and to providing resources needed by faculty, students, and staff to meet program objectives. Faculty, students, and administrators dance together in the study of nursing. Faculty support an environment that values the uniqueness of each person and sustains each person's unique way of living and growing in caring. This process requires trust, hope, courage, and patience. Because the purpose of nursing education is to study the discipline and practice of nursing, the nursed must be in the circle. The community created is that of persons living caring in the moment, each person valued as special and unique.

We have said in Chapter 1 that the domain of a discipline is that which its members assert. The statement of focus that directs the study of nursing from this theoretical perspective is that of nurturing persons as they live caring and grow in caring. The study of nursing is approached through the use of nursing situations. The knowledge of nursing resides in the nursing situation and is brought to life through study. The nursing situation is a shared lived experience in which the caring between the nurse and the one nursed enhances personhood, or the process of living grounded in caring. These situations, like the many cited in earlier chapters, become available for study through the use of story (recounting the situation in ways that convey the essence of the lived experience). These stories create anew the lived experience of caring between the nurse and the nursed, and bring to life the basic values described in Chapter One.

Story then becomes the method for studying and knowing nursing. Carper's (1978) four patterns of knowing serve as an organizing framework for asking epistemological questions of caring in nursing. Those patterns include personal, ethical, empirical, and aesthetic knowing. Each of these patterns come into play as one strives to understand the whole of the situation. Personal knowing centers on knowing and encountering self and other, empirical knowing addresses the science of caring in nursing, ethical knowing focuses on what "ought to be" in nursing situations, and aesthetic knowing is the integration and synthesis of all knowing as lived in a particular situation. The poem, "Intensive Care," a representation of a nursing situation, is given here to illustrate the organization of sample content.

INTENSIVE CARE

Did you see nurse that you can know me—
The part that is me, my mind and soul is in my eyes
These tubes that are everywhere—that is not me.
The one in my throat is the worst of all—
Now my whole being, the essence of me I
must reflect
through my hands but they are tied down,
movements
of my head but did you realize that
uncomfortable for me
or through my eyes and you do not notice them—
except once today during my bath.
You speak to me and look at the tubes—
Don't you know my thoughts are all over my face
Don't you realize your thoughts are on your face—
In your touch and your tone of voice.
I wrote a request on paper and you said "I'll take care
of it for you" your tone said "Why can't this
woman
Do anything for herself?"
You positioned your hand to count my pulse but I
Can't say you touched me—you wouldn't hold my
hand that I may touch you.

You walked in for the first time today with a grin
on your face but your mouth is now tight and
you grimaced a lot as you bathed me.
Don't you see nurse that you can know me—I'm not
a chart or tubes of medication, monitors or all
the other things you look at so intensely—I'm
more than that
I'm scared—just look in my eyes.

(S. Carr, 1991)

Carper's (1978) patterns of knowing offer a framework for organizing the content for studying this nursing situation.

Personal Knowing

Who are the nurse and nursed as caring persons in the moment?

How are the nurse and nursed expressing caring in this moment?

What is the meaning of this situation to the nurse and nursed in terms of present realities and future possibilities?

What is the meaning of vulnerability and mortality?

What is the value of intuition in practice?

Empirical Knowing

What nursing and related research exists on modes of communication, the meaning of presence in practice, touch, objectification, recovery of cardiac patients, technological caring, understanding the experience of fear and loneliness?

What factual knowledge is needed to be competent in this particular situation—e.g. knowledge of monitors, chest tubes, medications, cardiac care, diagnostic data?

Ethical Knowing

If nursing is practiced from the perspective of Nursing as Caring, what obligations are inherent in this situation?

How is the nurse demonstrating the value that all persons are caring? Respect for person-as-person? Interconnectedness?

What dilemmas are present in this story?

Aesthetic Knowing

How is the nursed supported to live dreams of living and growing in caring?

How could the nurse transcend the moment to create possibilities within this specific nursing situation?

What metaphors might express the meaning of this nursing situation?

Students studying this nursing situation are challenged to know the person as caring, as living caring uniquely in the moment, as having hopes and dreams for growing in caring, and being as whole or complete in the moment. The student is also challenged to know the nurse as caring person in the moment and to project ways of supporting the nurse as caring person.

Through the study of this situation, students and faculty identify a range of calls for nursing as well as nurturing responses. In this process, there is dialogue focused on knowing the nurse and nursed in the story as caring person. We would contribute the following as our knowing of the nursed as caring person. Through her honest expression of "I'm scared— just look in my eyes," we know her as living hope, honesty, and transcending fear through courage.

Calls for nursing might include a call to be known as caring person and a call to have interconnectedness recognized and affirmed. The nurse's response to these calls is individual and evolves from who one is as person and nurse. Therefore, the range of responses is multiple and varied— each reflecting the nurse's informed living of caring in the moment. Each nurturing response is focused on nurturing the person as he or she lives caring and expresses hopes and dreams for growing in caring.

If the nurse is responding to the call of the person for recognition and affirmation of interconnectedness, perhaps the nurse would express hearing this call by being present with the intention of knowing other as caring person. This may be communicated through active patience—giving the other time and space to be known; through touch which communicates respect and interconnectedness; through the nurse sharing who he or she is as caring person in this relationship—perhaps through tears as the resonance of commonality of this experience is known; through music or poetry if a shared love of these has been discovered.

Through dialogue, students and faculty openly engage in the study of nursing. The dialogue encourages and supports students and faculty to freely express who they are as person and nurse living caring through the re-presented story. It provides an opportunity to affirm values of self and discipline and to study how these values may be lived in practice. It is in this dialogue of nursing that faculty communicate their love for nursing. Time is needed for both faculty and students to reflect on the meaning of being a member of this discipline and more specifically, on the meaning of being a member of a discipline focused on nurturing persons as they live and grow in caring. Dialogue facilitates the integration of this understanding and is a key concept in present and future transformations of nursing education. Common engagement in dialogue as nursing stories are shared and studied is the way of being.

The story lived anew provides students the opportunity to participate in a lived experience of nursing and to create new possibilities. Since nursing can only occur through intentionality and authentic presence with the nursed, students and faculty share how they prepare to enter the world of the nursed, and how they come to understand that world. This process requires that students be encouraged to live fully their personhood. To facilitate such living, faculty support an environment in which students are free to choose and to express self in various ways. For example, perhaps the holistic understanding of a nursing situation would be expressed as aesthetic knowing through dance, poetry, music, painting, or the like. We view this process of education as critical to moral education. When students enter nursing situations to know other as living and growing in caring, they are living out the moral obligation that arises from the commitment to know person as caring. Here, then, is an expression of a dynamic view of morality in which caring is always lived in the moment.

In the study of the situation, *Intensive Care,* brought to the dialogue are personal experiences of being alone, being afraid, and being with someone and not being heard or seen as caring person. This personal knowing fosters human awareness of our connectedness and interdependence. In this context, the nurse does not study the empirics of cardiac pathology to understand a perceived deficit but rather to become competent in drawing forth the knowledge that is specific to knowing this person as whole in the moment. The nurse comes to know the person as living caring and growing in caring, situated within a particular set of circumstances, some of which the nurse knows explicitly. Each student entering the nursing situation will ask, "How can I nurture this person in living and growing in caring in this situation?" Because each nurse may hear calls for caring in many different ways, nursing responses are many and varied. For nursing faculty, openness to multiple possibilities presents a particular challenge and an opportunity to suspend entrenched patterns of teaching nursing.

Faculty and students study nursing together. Faculty join students in a constant search to discover the content and meaning of the discipline. Undoubtedly, this understanding of extant possibilities presents a different view of the role of teacher. Yet, it is a view that engenders the sort of humility essential to nursing for there is always more to know. Although past methods of teaching of nursing may have been comfortably structured through textbooks organized around medical science, faculty are now empowered to question what should be the focus of study in the discipline of nursing. Faculty are encouraged to take risks and let go of the familiar. The perspective that Nursing as Caring conveys—the fullness and richness of nursing—will allow faculty to willingly assume the risks inherent in a new way of guiding the study of nursing.

In teaching Nursing as Caring, faculty assist students to come to know, appreciate, and celebrate self and other as caring person. Mayeroff's *On Caring* (1971) provides a context for the generic knowing of self as caring. Through dyads or small groups, students share life situations in which they experienced knowing self and other as caring person. Mayeroff's caring ingredients (knowing, alternating rhythm, trust, honesty, hope, courage, humility, patience) also serve as a source for reflection as one asks "who am I as caring person?". As students engage this exercise, their emerging reflections begin to ground them as they grow in their understanding of person as they live and grow in caring. Students will also draw on the knowledge gleaned in the study of arts and humanities as they attempt to gain a deeper understanding of person. The process of knowing self and other as caring is lifelong. In an educational program grounded in Nursing as Caring, however, the focus on personal knowing (in the study of every nursing situation) provides a deliberate opportunity for greater knowing of self and other as caring person.

Students, as well as faculty, are in a continual search to discover greater meaning of caring as uniquely expressed in nursing. Journaling is an approach that facilitates this search. For example, in a special form of journaling, students actively dialogue with authors whose works they are reading and with the ideas expressed in their works. This process enhances the students' understanding of caring in nursing. Over time, students integrate and synthesize many ideas and create new understandings. Examination is another process to facilitate learning. From this theoretical perspective, essay examinations that present nursing situations provide opportunities for students to express their knowledge of nurturing persons living and growing in caring. Aesthetic projects also allow the student the opportunity to communicate understanding of a nursing situation. We would like to share with you a project from a course in which the students were asked to express the beauty of a nursing situation. In this nursing situation, the nurse, Michelle, shared her gifts of therapeutic touch and voice as expressions of caring for David in the moment, drawing on an earlier dialogue in which David told her of his love of meditation and the Ave Maria, she wrote:

AVE MARIA
and THERAPEUTIC TOUCH
FOR DAVID

"David, let me know your pain;
From fractured leg and heart,
Share with me your private hell.
Next to one who's far,
Far away in his own world:
Moaning, crying, weak.
What's it like to lie beside
One who cannot speak?

"Tell me David, what you do
To cancel out the sound;
Eliminate the smell of dung
In which your roommate's found?
Who can you complain about?
Are you worse off than he?
Tied to IV, traction lines
You cannot be free.

"David, I can see your pain.
Tell me where you are.
Tied in bed. Powerless.
From loved ones you're apart.
I can't move you from this place
To take your pain away.
But let me lay my hands on you
And sing to you today."

Ave Marie, gratia plena
Maria, gratia plena.
Ave dominus, dominus tecum.
Benedicta tu in mulieribus.
Et benedictus
Et benedictus, fructus ventris;

Implications for Nursing Education

Ventris tui, Jesu.
Ave Maria

I sang the song he loved and used
To meditate and flee,
Escape tormenting stimuli.
He needed to be freed,
To understand why he must bear
This trial, this hell, this pain,
I sang the tune; I touched with care
To give him peace again.

(Stobie, 1991)

Expressions of nursing such as this, which was partly sung, beautifully portray the living of caring between the nurse and the nursed and exemplify how caring enhances personhood. Faculty play a vital role in fostering in students the courage to take such risks. Faculty encourage self-affirmation in students, open, nonjudgmental dialogue, living the caring ideal in the classroom and development of the students' moral groundedness in caring (Boykin & Schoenhofer, 1990). Faculty also take the risk of sharing self through their stories of nursing. The sharing of nursing situations is, in essence, a sharing of our innermost core of common identity and forms a type of collegiality among those who are studying the discipline together.

How can faculty be supported to teach nursing in new ways? The administrator of the program fosters a culture in which the study of the discipline from the caring perspective, as presented here, can be achieved freely and fully. All actions of the dean are directed toward creating, maintaining, and supporting this goal. The theoretical assumptions ground the activities of the dean in both internal and external arenas of responsibility.

Internally, the administrator, faculty, staff, and students model commitment by creating an environment that fosters the knowing, living, and growing of persons in caring. The dean "ministers" by assuring that faculty, students, and staff are presented ongoing opportunities to know themselves ontologically as caring persons and professionals and to understand how caring orders their lives. Who we are as person influences who we are as student, colleague, nurse, scholar, and administrator. Therefore, attention must be directed to knowing self. Time must be devoted to knowing and experiencing our humanness.

The constant struggle to know self and other as caring person nourishes our knowing of the nursed. Through constant discovery of self, the other is also continually discovered. This culture sensitizes each person to ways of being with other that necessitate that each action reflect respect for person as person. Therefore, when issues are to be addressed, they are addressed openly and fully. Persons are encouraged to bring forth who they are so there is congruence between actions and feelings. Understanding each other's views is essential to the unfolding of this culture. Dialogue assists one to know the other's needs and desires, and to image oneself in the other's place. As such, the dean, faculty, staff, and students become skilled in the use of the caring ingredients, internalized as personally valid ways of expressing caring: knowing, alternating rhythms, trust, hope, courage, honesty, humility, and patience (Mayeroff, 1971).

Of utmost importance in fostering this culture are decisions regarding selection of faculty. Although many prospective faculty have a fairly traditional lens for the study of nursing (that is, the lens of medical science or frameworks borrowed from other disciplines), this actually becomes an insignificant factor in the process of selection. At the heart of choosing new faculty is knowing their passion for and love of nursing. A focus of the interview process is discerning the person's devotion to the discipline. It is our belief that this attitude, this love of nursing, is the music for the dancers in the circle. One way to know if prospective faculty love nursing is to ask them to share a significant story from practice. Having faculty share a story illuminates their conceptualization of the discipline. Many faculty who have not had the opportunity to teach nursing through an articulated nursing lens, can yet communicate nursing clearly through story.

Faculty are supported in their struggles to conceptualize nursing in a new way. Forums in which faculty come together and aesthetically re-present and share their nursing story is one strategy that effectively engages self and other in the knowing of nursing. It is also a wonderful way to orient faculty as to how to use nursing situations to teach nursing. Faculty support each other as colleagues in learning to teach nursing in a new way, in becoming expert in the practice of nursing education, and in living out the basic assumptions of this theory. This need for support holds true not only for faculty-faculty relationships but for all relationships. The comfort of faculty teaching nursing from the perspective of Nursing as Caring is enhanced as the value of knowing other as caring, as living our histories and as having special nursing stories to share is appreciated.

The administrator, faculty, and staff assist in fostering an environment that furthers the development of the students' capacity to care. Competency in caring is a goal of the educational process. Students are continually guided to know self and other as caring person as faculty and administrators model actions that reflect respect for person as person. Each student is known as caring person, as special and unique. Policies allow for consideration of individual situations and diverse possibilities. In this culture, the dean and faculty attempt to know the student as caring person and student of the discipline. The intention of the dean to know students in this way can be evident through invitations for regularly scheduled dialogue in which students share openly their conceptions about nursing. The administrator is truly with students to know them as caring persons and to hear from them their understanding of nursing as caring.

Externally, the dean "ministers" to faculty, students, and staff through securing resources necessary to accomplish program goals. The dean articulates to persons in the academic and broader community their role in the dance of nursing. The role of these persons is to provide resources such as scholarships, faculty development possibilities, learning resources, and research monies. Although this may be a primary responsibility of the dean by nature of the role, all persons in the circle share in this process by virtue of their commitment to nursing.

The administrator brings to the circle a skillful use of the caring ingredients. Alternating rhythms are used to understand and appreciate each person's unique contributions that support the achievement of program goals. For example, the budgetary process is essential to creating an environment that reflects the valuing of nursing. Commitment of the dean to securing resources necessary to accomplish the program goals drives the budget rather than the budget driving the commitment. The administrator's devotion to the discipline and to the basic assumptions of the theory direct all activities. The administrator makes decisions that reflect the basic beliefs of this theory. All decisions would ultimately be made from this standpoint: "What action should I take as administrator which would support the study of nursing as nurturing persons living in caring and growing in caring?"

What we have tried to suggest here is that every aspect of nursing education is grounded in the values and assumptions inherent in this theoretical focus. Thus, not only is the curriculum a direct expression of Nursing as Caring, but all aspects of program are similarly grounded.

REFERENCES

Boykin, A., & Schoenhofer, S. (1990). Caring in nursing: Analysis of extant theory. *Nursing Science Quarterly, 4,* 149–155.

Carper, B. (1978). Fundamental patterns of knowing in nursing. *Advances in Nursing Science, 1,* 13–24.

Carr, S. (1991). Intensive care. *Nightingale Songs,* P. O. Box 057563, West Palm Beach, FL 33405-7563, *2*(1).

Guralnik, D. (1976). *Webster's new world dictionary of the American language.* Cleveland: William Collings + World Publishing Co.

Mayeroff, M. (1971). *On caring.* New York: Harper & Row.

Nodding, N. (1988). An ethic of caring and its implications for institutional arrangement. *American Journal of Education, 97,* 215–230.

Stobie, M. (1991). Ave Maria and Therapeutic touch for David. *Nightingale Songs,* P. O. Box 057563, West Palm Beach, FL 33405-7563, *1*(3).

6

THEORY DEVELOPMENT AND RESEARCH

*I*n this concluding chapter, we will address our conception of nursing as human science and suggest directions and strategies for further development of the theory of Nursing as Caring. We initially introduced our perspective of nursing as discipline and profession in Chapter 1 and as a grounding context for the theory. As a discipline, nursing is a way of knowing, being, valuing, a way of living humanely, connected in oneness with others, living caring and growing in caring. The unity nursing offers is known in human experience through personal, empirical, ethical, and aesthetic realms.

Science has to do with knowing and that which is known. Philosophers of science are concerned with valid ways of knowing and ways of validating that which is known. Human science is described by scholars in various ways, each emphasizing particular values but all connecting to a common understanding that human science is concerned with knowing the world of human experience. A committed inquiry into human experience seems to call forth certain values related to the meaning of being human. Herein lies the fundamental difference between formal science and human science, as we perceive it. Formal science, that which is practiced in the natural sciences and other sciences that emulate them, is modeled on the structure of mathematics. Mathematics is a highly lawful science that has contributed enormous social benefits over time. However, formal science grounded in mathematics and languaged as calculus is an inappropriate approach to the study of person-as-person. A perspective that addresses the phenomenon of person-as-person is grounded in central values such as caring, freedom, and creativity. Methods to study person must be similarly grounded.

We have come to understand that valid ways of knowing nursing and legitimate warrants for nursing knowledge are discovered from within the study of nursing itself; that is, within the study of the nursing situation. The manner in which certain disciplines are conceptualized, especially those dealing in normative contexts, calls for a dialectical form of sciencing, comparing, and contrasting. However, coming to know nursing is a dialogical process—direct engagement with the "word of nursing." Nursing science must be contextual; the decontextualized methodology of formal science, while essential for certain disciplines, cannot reveal direct knowledge of nursing. Because of the nature of nursing, nursing science must permit intentionality, intimacy, mutuality, and particularity.

Human science has understanding as its goal, with the definite expectation that understanding is in the moment only (Watson, 1988; Van Manen, 1990). In addition, the nature of nursing praxis does not require knowledge for the purpose of control, but for enlightenment, moment-to-moment and reflectively. The nurse seeks knowledge neither to control one's own behavior nor that of the nursed. If it were otherwise, the nurse would become his or her own prisoner, and would relate to the other as dominator rather than caring nurse. The concept of the hermeneutic circle informs our understanding of the nature of nursing as a human science. This circle of understanding, really a sphere more than a unidimensional circle, is an heuristic device which directs our attention. As attention pauses at any aspect of the nursing situation, we must attend to other aspects and to the whole of the nursing situation to create useful understanding. One hermeneutist has pointed out that the circle brings *us* further along, not the issue at hand (Droysen, 1988). This distinction points to the human science position that understanding is not constituted through analysis of facts but through dialogue with text and context. That is, what moves within the circle is the seeker, rather than that which is sought, so that many aspects are illuminated in context, and understanding grows. The hermeneutic circle requires that what we note in our inquiry remains contextualized, developing "new and ever new circles" (Boeckh, 1988). This is in contrast to normal science that requires an external referent for objects of study in order to avoid circular thinking. Heidegger (1988), for example, contrasts the vicious circle of normal science (tautology) with the circle of hermeneutic understanding: ". . . in the circle is hidden a positive possibility of the most primordial kind of knowing" (p. 225). We would propose that valid knowing in nursing is that which is known from within the circle.

While the work of several scholars has influenced our understanding (e.g., Gadamer, 1989; Van Manen, 1990; Ray, in press; Reeder, 1988), Macdonald's (1975) interpretation from the field of humanistic education is especially meaningful. He explains hermeneutic knowing methodologically as "circular rather than linear in that the interpretation of meaning in hermeneutic understanding depends on a reciprocal relation" (p. 286) rather than on a fixed normative reference point. The hermeneutic circle models the idea of reciprocal relation, but Macdonald goes further to call for a self-reflective science that will "transcend problems of monological and hermeneutic meaning" (p. 287). The nature of nursing as expressed in the Nursing as Caring theory is a reciprocal relation, one characterized by its grounding in person as caring, and as persons connected in oneness in caring. Sciencing in nursing from this perspective must go beyond linearity to encompass the dialogic circling involved in the nursing situation. This places the discipline of nursing among the human sciences, and calls for methods of inquiry that assure the circle or dialogue, and further, fully accommodate that which can be known of nursing.

Nursing is properly catalogued as one of the human sciences for many reasons. The most basic reason is that the discipline and the disciplined practice of nursing directly involves persons in the fullness of their humanness. From our perspective, this means person as caring. Person as caring implies person in community, connected in oneness with others and with the universe, person freely choosing the living of values which are expressions of caring. This nursing ontology requires an epistemology consonant with human science values and methods. To know of, through and with nursing necessitates methods and techniques that honor freedom, creativity, and interconnectedness.

In Chapter 4, we asserted that nursing knowledge is created and discovered within and from within the nursing situation. (Nursing situation, you may recall, is understood as a shared lived experience in which the caring between the nurse and the one nursed enhances personhood.) Therefore, because the locus of nursing inquiry is the nursing situation, the systematic study of nursing calls for a new methodology that recognizes that fact.

Certainly, we acknowledge that something useful for nursing can be learned through existing methodologies, from both natural and human science traditions. For example, an experimental design can produce information about the effectiveness of a given clinical technique within a specified range of use (e.g., placement of an oral thermometer). Such information can be important and useful to the work of the nurse and useful to the client of nursing. It tells us nothing, however, of nursing. In fact, the central tenet underlying measurement in normal science directly contradicts the central tenet of human science: created versus creating. Thus, the fullness of the nursing situation is not amenable to study by measurement techniques. Yet, aspects of the nursing situation can be abstracted and studied as variables in relation to other variables. This does not, however, yield knowledge of the nursing situation in its fullest. At best, measurement approaches can call attention to an aspect so that it can be considered within the unfolding.

Phenomenology, on the other hand, offers an example of an orientation and methodology that more closely approximates what is needed in a nursing method of inquiry. Phenomenology is an orientation toward inquiry that may be actualized through any one of a number of generic approaches, but is generally understood as the study of lived experience (e.g., Van Manen, 1990; Oiler, 1986). When the phenomenon conceptualized for study is representative of the nursing situation, nursing may be known. That is, new nursing knowledge may eventuate. New understanding of the meaning of the shared lived experience of caring between nurse and nursed enhancing personhood can be created.

Yet, for the purposes of nursing, phenomenology also has its limits. For example, when phenomena which have been abstracted from a nursing situation are selected for study (that is, when phenomena are taken out of context), results of the inquiry cannot generate knowledge of nursing proper. For example, the understanding that comes in developing a description of the essential structure of what it is like for a nurse to be called to nurse informs us about nurses, but not about nursing directly. Similarly, an exquisite phenomenological description of what it is like for a person to live grieving is helpful in understanding the person. However, it should not be mistaken for knowledge of nursing, but knowledge which illuminates the study of nursing when taken back to the full context of the nursing situation. Further, the various phenomenologies in the literature come from frames of reference that are not nursing (e.g., existential psychology or educational psychology), and thus impose a "silent" borrowed framework when used to study nursing.

Is this drawing too fine a line? And is it really important to press the issue of nursing knowledge versus knowledge of and for nurses? The answers to these questions are probably found in one's concept of nursing as a field of knowledge (discipline) and a human service (profession). It seems that nursing and nurses have suffered significantly over the years with this dilemma. Is it possible to have a sense of self as nurse without a concomitant sense of nursing as a discipline which is more than tacit and to which one is committed? Students of nursing and practitioners alike have abundant opportunities to acquire a sense of self as nurse. Yet why is it that many programs of nursing education (at all levels) do not convey a sense of nursing as a discipline? The answer may lie in those conducting the programs, who have experienced training for practice and education in disciplines other than nursing and without explicit education in the discipline of nursing.

From the perspective of Nursing as Caring, with its grounding in person as caring and nursing as a discipline, the distinctions implied in this question of "does it really matter" are of central importance. Nurses in practice, education, and administration continue to address nursing primarily in terms of "what nurses do," (e.g., nursing "interventions") and most nursing research seems to derive from that perspective as well. Without a clearly articulated understanding of the focus of the discipline, it has been extremely difficult to organize and structure nursing knowledge in ways that facilitate the development of the discipline. In this book, we have offered a theory, Nursing as Caring, as one expression of that focus, languaged in terms that communicate the essence of nursing.

Nursing knowledge is knowledge of nurturing persons living caring and growing in caring within shared lived experiences in which the caring between nurse and nursed enhances personhood. Furthering nursing knowledge requires methods that can illuminate the central phenomenon of the discipline. The development of such a methodology is, as we see it, the next major effort to be undertaken in the development of the theory. In this regard, we envision a fully adequate methodology that would include a phenomenological aspect which goes beyond description to a hermeneutical process, within an action research orientation. That is, what seems to be needed is a methodology that would permit the study of nursing meaning as it is being co-created in the lived experience of the nursing situation. Supplemental methods could continue to include traditional phenomenological and hermeneutic work with texts describing particular nursing situations. Nurses who are interested in developing knowledge of techniques or modes of expressing caring would continue to use traditional methods of formal and human science for these kinds of nursing-related questions.

The development of methods of nursing inquiry appropriate to the study of the theory, Nursing as Caring, is in a formative stage. We understand to a considerable extent the limitations of existing modes of inquiry, and have a growing sense of what will be required of a new methodology. Nursing scholars are working to develop methods to illuminate the fullness of nursing. Examples of that work which has encouraged our efforts include that by Parker (1993), Swanson-Kauffman (1986), Parse (1990), and Ray (Wallace, 1992). The work of these scholars demonstrates that the development of nursing ways of inquiry is important and that a search has begun. As we have come to understand the concept of human science, our understanding of nursing has been enriched. Like most of our contemporaries in nursing, we were trained in the often unarticulated assumptions of natural science. And we have travelled the road familiar to many nursing scholars, the road of expertise in objectification and quantification. Along that road, we began to notice the trivialization of cherished nursing ideas like presence, touch, relationship, knowing, and caring. Resisting the temptation to abandon the journey, we each persevered in a commitment to nursing as something which mattered, something involving intimate, personal, caring relationships. Discovering, inventing, and creating a new methodology is an important dream and we are committed to continuing this aspect of theory development.

Nursing as Caring is a transformational model for all arenas. Nursing practice, nursing service organization, nursing education, and nursing inquiry require a full understanding of nursing as nurturing persons living caring and growing in caring, and these underlying assumptions:

- Persons are caring by virtue of their humanness.
- Persons are caring, moment to moment.
- Persons are whole or complete in the moment.
- Personhood is a process of living grounded in caring.
- Personhood is enhanced through participating in nurturing relationships with caring others.
- Nursing is both a discipline and profession.

With these transformations, the fullness of nursing will be realized and we will grow in our understanding of self and other as caring persons connected in oneness.

REFERENCES

Boeckh, P. (1988). Theory of criticism. In K. Mueller-Vollmer (Ed.), *The hermeneutics reader*. New York: Continuum.

Droysen, J. (1988). The investigation of origins. In K. Mueller-Vollmer (Ed.). *The hermeneutics reader*. New York: Continuum, pp. 124–126.

Gadamer, H. (1989). *Truth and method.* New York: Crossroad Publishers.

Heidegger, M. (1988). Understanding and interpretation. In K. Mueller-Vollmer (Ed.), *The hermeneutics reader.* New York: Continuum, pp. 221–228.

Macdonald, J. (1975). Curriculum and human interests. In W. Pinar, *Curriculum theorizing: The reconceptualists.* Berkeley: McCutchan Publishers.

Oiler, C. (1986). Phenomenology: The method. In P. Munhall & C. Oiler (Eds.), *Nursing research: A qualitative perspective.* Norwalk, CT: Appleton-Century-Crofts.

Parker, M. (1993). *Living nursing values in nursing practice.* Paper presented at 7th Annual Conference of the Southern Research Association, Birmingham, AL, February 18, 1993.

Parse, R. (1990). Parse's research methodology with an illustration of the lived experience of hope. *Nursing Science Quarterly, 3,* 9–17.

Ray, M. A. (in press). The richness of phenomenology: Phenomenologic-hermeneutic approaches. In J. Morse (Ed.), *Critical issues in qualitative research. A contemporary dialogue.* Newbury Park, CA: Sage.

Reeder, F. (1988). Hermeneutics. In B. Sarter (Ed.), *Paths to Knowledge.* New York: National League for Nursing.

Swanson-Kauffman, K. (1986). A combined qualitative methodology for nursing research. *Advances in Nursing Science, 8*(3), 58–69.

Van Manen, M. (1990). *Researching lived experience.* London, Ontario: State University of New York Press.

Wallace, C. (1992). *A conspiracy of caring: The meaning of the client's experience of nursing as the promotion of well-being.* Unpublished master's thesis, College of Nursing, Florida Atlantic University.

Watson, J. (1988). *Nursing: Human science and human care. A theory of nursing.* New York: National League for Nursing.

INDEX

Index

Nurse administrator, 60–61
  budget decisions, 63–64
  and calls for nursing, 61–62, 68
  nursing situation, 62–63
  relationship to direct care,
    60–61
Nursed as caring person, 22
Nursing: A Social Policy Statement
    (American Nurses
    Association), 12
Nursing as Caring
  as stabilizer of organization,
    65–66
  discipline and profession,
    nursing as, 10–16
  educational program grounded
    in, 81
  ideas related to, 3–16
  ideologies/cognitive frameworks
    not congruent with, 52
  nurse administrator decisions,
    61
  persons as caring, perspective
    of, 3–10
  transformational model, 98
  theory, xiii–xiv, 21–29
Nursing Development Conference
    Group, xiv
  *Concept Formalization in Nursing:
    Process and Product,* 11, 14
Nursing Diagnosis movement,
    52–53, 55–56, 57
*Nursing: Human Science and Human
    Care. A Theory of Nursing*
    (Watson), 6, 28, 92
"Nursing on the caring edge;
    Metaphorical vignettes"
    (Watson), 36
"Nursing Process" (Orlando),
    52–53, 56
"Nursing research and social
    control: Alternative models of
    science that emphasize

understanding and
    emancipation (Allen), 13
Nursing situation, 15–16, 23, 28,
    33–40, 81
  and administration, nursing,
    62–63
  education, nursing, 74, 77–78,
    81
  persons with altered levels of
    consciousness, 35–36
  re-presentation of via art forms,
    37
  shared lived experience, 35,
    37–40, 48–49, 56
  study of, 77–78
  theory development, 94

Oiler, C.
  "Phenomenology: The method,"
    95
On Caring (Mayeroff), 4–6, 8, 45,
    58, 80–81, 84
"On dialogue" (Bohm), 63
Orem, D. E.
  Nursing: Concepts of Practice, 28,
    29
  Self-Care Deficit Theory of
    Nursing, 28, 29
Organization
  hierarchical model of, 65–66
  stabilizer, Nursing as Caring as,
    65
Orlando, I.
  *The Dynamic Nurse-Patient
    Relationship,* 52
  Nursing Process approach, 52–53

Packard, S. A.
  "The dilemma of nursing
    science: Current quandaries
    and lack of direction," 12
Parenthood, nursing profession as,
    27–28

15.95